Pregnancies Collected

Pregnancies Collected

Stories for Every Month of Your Pregnancy

Cheryl J. Hancock

Writers Club Press
San Jose New York Lincoln Shanghai

Pregnancies Collected
Stories for Every Month of Your Pregnancy

Writers Club Press
an imprint of iUniverse.com, Inc.

For information address:
iUniverse.com, Inc.
5220 S 16th, Ste. 200
Lincoln, NE 68512
www.iuniverse.com

ISBN: 0-595-19005-7

Printed in the United States of America

Dedication

This book is dedicated to my babies Mara and Derek who caused me to seek a book like this one. I am blessed to have been pregnant twice and to have two healthy and beautiful children.

Epigraph

How amazing, you
round, swollen belly
you shape shifter,
safe keeper.
Only my imagination
sees inside to your
hidden treasure of
tiny fingers and toes,
floating smiles and
silent cries…
as I suffer the
twinges and fuddles
brought of the swell.
Soon brings metamorphosis,
me and little one…
I a mother become,
little one, a child,
and what of that
the stories do tell!
How amazing, we!

Cheryl J. Hancock

Contents

Acknowledgements

This book would not have been possible without the generosity of the hundreds of women who graciously offered their personal pregnancy stories. A great thanks goes to all of these women (and the dads too) and their contributions to the following pages. All of the stories are true and very few names were changed for privacy purposes.

Also, thanks to my husband and children, who thought I was attached to my computer, for having patience with me during the time consuming writing of this book.

Introduction

Why I Wrote This Book

When I discovered I was pregnant with my second child, not only did I begin crying with hysterical joy, but immediately I began trying to remember every detail of my first pregnancy. That automatic reaction to seek the information of what I would endure calmed me since my first pregnancy was primarily uneventful. The most I suffered was only one or two tinges of pain my midwife regarded as my uterus stretching. Other than that, I had a pretty normal pregnancy, or so I thought. I also thought my second one couldn't be any worse than my first. Boy, was I wrong. I had no idea what I was in for, for it was nothing like my first pregnancy at all. I soon realized after her birth that no pregnancy could be considered normal.

Constantly bombarded with sickness, discomfort, sudden and overwhelming weight gain, and fatigue, my second was everything else my first pregnancy wasn't. I worried if such differences meant my baby would be affected or if I wasn't doing something right. I'd ask others if they had experienced the same or similar situations with their bodies, and I'd read the pages of birth books over and over looking for some hint of explanation I might have missed. I also began to panic. I worried I was going to get bigger the second time, that I would get even more stretch marks, and that my body would ever be the same again afterward. Ugh!

Because I was so worried and constantly agonizing over the differences I was experiencing, I thought it might be comforting if I knew and could compare what others were experiencing. I had many new questions and never enough answers. I also found myself dealing with sometimes funny and sometimes difficult issues, from telling my son about my new pregnancy to dealing with in-laws and other family members.

So, the idea of this book stemmed from wondering what everyone else who had been pregnant was going through and if their pregnancies were anything like mine. During my pregnancy, everyone had advice to give, stories to share, and old wives tales to tell. At times, I was more curious than irritated at this unsolicited wisdom, so I thought I'd collect this information moms and grandmoms (and dads, too!) were so willing to share.

And, here it is, for you and every other wonderfully pregnant woman: a collective of experiences at every stage of pregnancy: examples of horrors, pleasures, and some hysterical moments typical of what I discovered to be a "normal" pregnancy, since there is no such thing. But remember, this book is for comfort value only; for the formal doctor's discussion, I recommend seeking books such as *What to Expect When You're Expecting*, and other such titles.

Cheryl J. Hancock

Chapter I

The First Month I

"Death and taxes and childbirth! There's never any convenient time for any of them!"

Margaret Mitchell, "Gone with the Wind"

You're Pregnant!!!

Pregnancy is typically most like a nine-month long roller coaster ride: non-stop ups and downs and endless twists and turns. Each month is different from the next, sometimes scary and other times exciting and emotionally, if not physically, exhausting. One second you're on top of the world and the next you're free-falling into a nervous panic, and sometimes screaming the whole way. If you feel overwhelmed, you're not alone.

The first month of pregnancy is usually the time of discovery, and how you find out you are pregnant can be an experience in itself. Though some do, not all women immediately intuitively "know" or feel any symptoms. This initial discovery can be as frustrating as many of the symptoms that will inevitably come along with it. As you will read, each woman has a different discovery experience from incorrect pregnancy tests to no or completely diverse symptoms.

My first pregnancy was largely uneventful, and I was two months pregnant when I first found out. I had not missed my cycle, but my breasts were very tender. Not having a doctor, I talked to some colleagues and found out about a midwife who had a great reputation. She was less expensive than a regular OB/GYN, and I was told she was extremely caring. (Choosing a doctor is another issue.)

When the test came back as positive, I became worried if the beer I had drunk or anything else I had done like working out at the gym or smoking cigarettes had affected the baby. However, my midwife encouraged me that nature had a way of taking care of a fetus who has not yet been discovered.

With my second child, I found out very early since I was eager to have another baby. However, before my discovery, I had an X-ray at the chiropractor for my back trouble and was scared it may have affected the little fetus. Many of the women you will meet in this chapter have had similar experiences.

With both pregnancies, I had little or no morning sickness. However, with my second, I did have a horrible taste in my mouth for a long time, and since I detested the taste and smell of cigarettes, I was very moody from quitting smoking. Some women experience morning, noon, and night sickness, all differently, and sometimes suffer painfully.

The first month of a pregnancy can be a traumatic or uneventful experience, depending upon your body's decision and current condition. If you don't already have a dependable OB/GYN or midwife, you will need to choose one. There are many differences in the two, and you may feel more comfortable with one doctor over another. Your doctor may decide to have you complete a physical examination if you are a new patient. Your age and health history may be important factors in this exam process as well as in your symptoms.

You may be considered high risk because of age, handicap, or health condition. You also may be worried about a recent x-ray exam, prescription drug, or alcoholic drink you may have had. Maybe you had difficulty becoming pregnant, have had a miscarriage or took fertility drugs. You may have been waiting for and agonizing over this exact moment your whole life. You may be feeling guilt, fear, excitement, anxiety, or profound happiness.

Once you've discovered your new found condition, you'll have to decide when and how to announce this great news. I'll never forget when my husband called to tell his mother I was pregnant. I could hear her scream on the phone from excitement from three feet away. Sometimes it can be a touchy decision, especially if you've had a prior miscarriage and aren't sure you want to tell anyone so soon.

Whatever your situation, here are some words of wisdom, true stories, remedies and old wives tales women have openly shared for you and your first month of pregnancy. Some you may find truly funny and others may touch you deeply.

Alcohol and Cigarettes

When I first suspected that I might be pregnant, I quit smoking cold turkey. There was no question about it. I wouldn't do anything to hurt my baby. What I didn't know was that by quitting so abruptly, my blood pressure went through the roof. My doctor said that because I had been smoking for so long and because I smoked at least a half a pack of cigarettes a day, that the baby and I would be safer instead if I cut down gradually and steadily. I got down to one or two cigarettes in two or three days. That's not perfect, and I'm not proud to say that I smoked at all during pregnancy. However, I am glad that I had so much positive encouragement from my doctor. I could have lost my baby due to my blood pressure being so high when I thought I was doing the right thing.

Krystal, Canada.

Even before I found out I was pregnant, cigarette smoke began to smell really bad, and I had decided to cut way back toward quitting altogether. Not a week or so later, I found out I was pregnant and realized the reason for the smell and figured that was Mother Nature's signal. That's when I put the cigarettes down for good. For about three weeks, I was a total witch. I didn't speak to my husband for two weeks because he irritated me. Once the nicotine was out of my system, I looked back on the hardest two weeks of my life. I also apologized to my husband who graciously accepted and told me I wasn't "that bad."

Jane, 27, Daytona, FL.

Announcements

When I found out I was pregnant, I didn't know how I would tell our families. My friend told me what she had heard someone else do, and I knew my husband and my families were going to be together for the holiday. I put a T-shirt on my 3 year-old little boy that said "I'm a big brother," and I sent him into the room when everyone was together. You should have seen the reaction on the faces! They were all excited for us, and we have a story to tell for generations.

Michelle, 31. Mississippi.

I had always wanted a baby, but my husband wasn't quite ready. I had been pleading to have him not use protection. Well, when I found out, I was only about three weeks along, but I had had a pregnancy test the previous month, proving how much I wanted this to happen. I went to a volunteer women's clinic dedicated to helping young women decide to keep their babies just to get a professional test done. They made me watch a video on abortion (I definitely wanted my baby). It wasn't fun until she came out with the good news! I floated all the way home. When my husband came home, I handed him a folded paper that looked like another bill. When he opened it, he read about the good news and saw where the nurse had signed it. He didn't speak much until he called his mother with the good news!

Sheryl, 26, Jacksonville, FL

My husband and I weren't sure how to tell our parents that we were pregnant, so instead, we gift-wrapped a rattle and a pacifier in little boxes. We called both sets of parents for dinner one evening and gave one present to each couple after dinner. They immediately realized they were going to be grandparents!

Celia, New York.

I waited a while before I finally told my parents that I was pregnant. After my first ultrasound, I scanned the picture of what looked like a little, round blob and made a card with Print Master software on my computer. When they saw the card, their faces told their surprise.

Sylvia, 29, Oklahoma.

Body Changes

I couldn't stand the smell of soup or coffee anymore, two things I really love.

Jean, 68, Georgia.

In my first month of pregnancy, I noticed a sudden change in my ability to breath properly, and I developed allergies I had never had before. My doctor said I could take the plain, little, red Sudafed pills, but he really wanted me to rough it out. He also recommended a nose spray that is saline solution only called Ayr or something like it. It worked well at night when I needed to clean my sinuses to sleep. For itchy-watery eyes, I was given eye drops with an antihistamine, which worked wonders.

Samantha, 21, California.

I knew immediately that I was pregnant the second time. I think I wanted it so bad that I just "knew" I had to be. I also began to gain weight, and smells began to bother me. I never was sick but very sensitive to all smells, especially the laundry detergent isle at the grocery store.

Mandy, 29. Seattle.

My breasts have always been sensitive, but when I got pregnant, it seemed that even putting on a bra made my breasts respond. They itched a lot too. It was great when it came to sex, but at other times, I hated it.

Katy, Ohio.

Choosing a Doctor

I had chosen a doctor that I really wanted to see but they wouldn't see me unless I had a positive pregnancy test. I had already missed my first period, so I made an appointment to take a test, took the urine specimen to the doctor, and it came out negative. By the time I was supposed to have my second period, I knew I was definitely pregnant. I took another urine specimen, and it came back negative again. The doctor didn't think I was pregnant, so he wouldn't see me. By the time I did test positive, I was almost 4 months pregnant, and I was seeing another doctor. I was very naive then, and I don't think doctors do that anymore. However, I recall thinking how I didn't receive prenatal care for those first months because the doctor wanted a positive test. I just didn't have enough of the hormone that causes a positive test.

Marie, 49. Dayton, Ohio.

Choosing a doctor is important because not all doctors are the same, and not all women want to have the basic OB/GYN or hospital birth. I wanted to have a natural childbirth, meaning no drugs or epidurals, and couldn't afford a regular doctor, so I decided to go with a midwife. Midwives are very experienced nurses with specialization in childbirth and a varying number of years of education. I enjoyed seeing my midwife who was always very friendly and personable. I remember seeing one of the doctors in the same building when my midwife wasn't available, and he rushed our visit and wasn't very talkative. I also enjoyed thinking I might actually give birth without medications!!

Theresa, 30. Oklahoma City.

I was four weeks along when I found out about my pregnancy, and I went to see an OB/GYN. I had bleeding soon after, and he told me it was "polyps." When the bleeding continued almost daily, he said it was a cervical infection. He said, "Use this cream." The bleeding continued again almost daily and in my 15th week, my husband went with me insisting on a sonogram. The doctor took four days to call me with the results showing a low placenta. I had to self-educate by reading books and other material, which only scared me more. In my 17th week, I switched doctors and found one who made sure I understood what was happening and that the condition usually corrects itself. That's what happened, and with a little compassion and understanding from my new doctor, I felt better about what I thought was an unnecessarily scary pregnancy.

Natasha, 25. Iowa.

Diet

With my first child, I gained over 50 pounds. I stopped counting after a certain point. So, when I found out about my second pregnancy, I immediately thought of the previous weight gain and decided that wasn't going to happen this time. I put myself on a great diet, one I discovered through a friend who was on it because of her diabetes. I ate less sugar and fat, drank skim milk, and cut out junk foods that aren't good for anyone anyway. I actually lost some weight in my first month and never gained more than 25 pounds the whole way through.

Janet, 31, Gainesville, FL.

When I noticed the first five pounds, I blew it off to over-eating or indulging. When I noticed the second five pounds, I knew something was up. I know my body really well and had been pregnant once already. I took a pregnancy test around the fifth week, when I was a couple of days late for my period, and I knew instantly. With my second baby, everything happened sooner, the weight gain, the sore breasts, the bloating. I knew I had to catch my weight before it escalated, which would be easy for me, but I began to feel like I was starving all the time with hunger pains every hour. I needed a muzzle. Why does pizza have to taste so good?!

Rose, 29, Alabama.

Due Date

I couldn't remember the exact day or night we conceived, but I knew I wasn't due in February with my son. When I found out about the pregnancy, I was 4 weeks pregnant, but at my first sonogram, the doctor said I was further along. I chose the due date around January 21st, and the doctor said February 16th. My son was born January 26th at 7 pounds, 12 ounces. Sometimes you just know.

Kelsey, Arizona.

I was trying to plan my pregnancy leave by my doctor's due date and was unsure the doctor actually had it right. I was really confused about how they used the date of the last day of your last period and add nine months, and one nurse mentioned something about counting backwards a couple of months. My due date came out to be January 15, but when my doctor did a sonogram at three months, he changed it due to the baby's size. My due date became December 28. I had the baby on December 27, and my pregnancy leave just had to be then no matter what I had already put in for.

Candis, 40, Tampa, FL.

Exercise

I think more emphasis should be placed on doing Kegel exercises (that I only did sporadically). These exercises help strengthen the uterus and the muscles around it, so you will have less problems with bladder control after pregnancy. I also should say that my husband and I were told some gentle stretches that he could do for me, if I preferred, for the peritoneal tissue to prevent tearing during delivery. Ask your doctor about these. They're fun.

Franlie, 37, Guelph, ON.

I was so happy to hear from my doctor that I could keep exercising when I became pregnant. I was always afraid that I would gain excess weight and the muscle tone I had would disappear. I never wanted to end up substantially heavier after my pregnancy. I was told to keep doing aerobics and weight training as long as I didn't strain myself too much or start anything new that I wasn't already used to. Then, the doctor said as I move further along in my pregnancy, that I would eventually be required to alter my workout, such as not lying on my back after four months and lowering the intensity gradually. I worked out until I was 8 months pregnant when I became so tired that I was spending the little bit of energy I did have at the gym. Then, I enjoyed sleeping all the more.

Tracy, 28, Dallas, TX.

High Risk

I have always been a diabetic, well, at least since I was about 12 years old. So, when I found out I was pregnant, I was very excited but also nervous. I managed my diabetes with my diet, and I exercised and took good care of myself. I pretty much knew that I would have to treat my body the same and be extra aware of any other symptoms I noticed. My doctor wanted a complete work-up when I tested positive to be sure of where I was physically. The tests came out fine and my first month was good. I had some morning sickness, but not enough to keep me from eating or staying on my diet.

Evelyn, 30, San Diego, CA.

When I was pregnant with my first daughter, I found out early that I was RH-. Let's say that my blood type is A and my husband's blood type is B. Since they are not the same, the baby could end up being B like my husband's. When the mother and baby's blood types don't match, the mother's body may try to attack the fetus as an intruder like the flu or something. You receive a needle in your hip at 26 weeks, of a drug called Ro-gram, and the problem is basically solved. You also get another shot after delivery to save further pregnancies. When I heard about this, I found it very confusing and went to others to try to understand. This is the explanation I received from my doctor as well as friends. It can be a very scary process to undergo unless your doctor handles the issue well.

Deanne, Lafayette, LA.

Every time I would visit my doctor, he would quiz me on my blood type. If I were ever in an accident, I would need to know what to tell emergency physicians. This is a good thing for doctors to do with RH factor patients.

Natalie, 25, Paris, TX.

At 4 weeks pregnant, my doctor found 3 very large fibroids in my uterus as well as a large number of little ones. I was labeled high-risk from the beginning, but had no complications. The only complaint I had was the pain they caused. The fibroids are made up of muscle and blood, and they cause a great deal of cramping. The first trimester was the worst for me and was like having tremendous menstrual cramps, but that subsided after about 3 months. The only other thing after that was my size. I was in maternity clothes at 10 weeks because the tumors were so large, and at 7 months I finally looked somewhat normal in size.

Gretchan, 32, Wichita, KS.

Initial Discovery

I found out I was pregnant because my face broke out in pimples very badly. I usually get two or three before my periods. It seemed that by the time I was two weeks late, I had 100 zits on my face. The pregnancy test confirmed it. My skin continued to get really bad, and then I developed cystic acne. I used topical erythromycin, but that was no help. Now I try to deal with the scars and pock marks on my once clear face.

Barbara, 27, Thornton, CO.

I was three months pregnant before I found out, and it was only because my husband made me go to the doctor for testing to determine why I was experiencing extreme shortness of breath. I have never had regular periods, more like three or four a year. Thankfully the technician at the x-ray lab insisted on a pregnancy test before doing the chest x-ray. I had insisted it wasn't necessary because I'd never heard of shortness of breath being a symptom of pregnancy. I got the call with the positive results, and I was so stunned I could hardly breathe!

Franlie, 37, Guelph, ON.

I was 24, living with my parents, and finishing a Master's degree when I found myself pregnant. I didn't tell my parents for a month and a half, which was very hard. When they found out they cried and cried. I found it hard not to be able to talk to my mother about her pregnancy experience while I was pregnant, but she did not want to face the fact that I was pregnant. Although my parents eventually came around, I did not talk to my mother about pregnancy, hers or mine, until the end. They were just not happy about it. Not being able to share my feelings with the important people in my life who were mad and sad was very difficult.

Rosalie, 27. Montreal, Quebec.

My marriage was in serious trouble, and we had only had sex one time in 10 months. That's when I got pregnant. I had to get out of the marriage, and I told him I didn't love him anymore or want to be married. We had tried counseling against his wishes, and it just wasn't working. Now that I was pregnant, I felt terrible, like my life was over and the baby's as well. My first month was the hardest, when I cried the most thinking that I couldn't bring a baby into a failed marriage or into a single family home. I struggled through my pregnancy and in the end, fell in love with her and myself. I also say God helped me through the ordeal because we are happy and healthy, and her father has come around too.

Tammy, Oakland, NJ.

My husband and I found out about my pregnancy at about three weeks. All I did for the next three days was cry and feel sad. I guess it was because I thought that I would have more time with my husband, career, new house, etc. The pregnancy wasn't unplanned, just three years early.

Lucy, Ontario.

Initial Examinations

My periods had been irregular before I got pregnant. When I went for my first prenatal exam, I was nine weeks pregnant according to my last period. However, the doctor was concerned because I was only measuring about six weeks, so she scheduled a sonogram. The technician immediately found the "pregnancy sac," but we could not see anything in the sac. The doctor came and performed a vaginal sonogram with the same results. He told us that either the pregnancy was very early, about 5 weeks along, or that I had a blighted ovum, a condition where the egg does not develop. I sat in the room and cried feeling in limbo. I had so many questions about the brownish spotting I had been experiencing and about the blighted ovum. My doctor told me there was a 50/50 chance the egg would develop and had me schedule another sonogram 10 days later. I couldn't watch television commercials about babies or look at babies in the stores. I turned to my Bible and read Psalm 139 for comfort. I spent hours on the Internet trying to find out more about pregnancy sacs, their measurements and blight ovums. At the next sonogram, we immediately saw "something" there! The egg had developed, and we could see its tiny heartbeat. We found out that I was 7 weeks pregnant.

Christie, 26. Austin, Texas.

Morning (noon and evening) Sickness

I was one of the lucky ones because I had no morning sickness at all. But my appetite never seemed to be satisfied. I had to eat every 2 to 3 hours because I was so hungry.

Joanne, Boise, ID.

I had terrible morning sickness in my first month of pregnancy, which was the initial clue that I was pregnant. I spoke to my mother and friends about what would help me, and I found the common cure to be eating saltine crackers. Someone also told me to drink Sprite. I was told not to get out of bed quickly and not to shower or drive on an empty stomach. I found that sometimes just giving into the sickness was helpful as well because at least then I wasn't sick anymore.

Gina, 33. Pennsylvania.

Morning sickness plagued me for almost the first six months of my pregnancy. I puked almost every day. Back then, the doctors used to give you shots for it, although I can't remember what the shot was. They were afraid my baby would have a low birth weight because I kept throwing up, so I had the shot two or three times. It didn't help me at all. I couldn't even put my hands in dirty water to rinse a sponge without vomiting. Then years later, I found out the shots they gave me later caused birth defects.

Darlene, 47, New Milford, NJ.

Someone suggested I try sipping Pedialyte, you know the stuff you give sick babies, and it really helped my nausea. It was also very soothing on my stomach. Pedialyte doesn't taste very great, but if you can get past that, it will help re-hydrate your body. Also, I was told about Ginger Root Tea, which also worked well for me. I just took the root and finely chopped a tablespoon or so to put in a tea infuser in a cup of boiling water for five minutes or so. My nausea subsided so that I could eat, which was what I needed at that point.

Rosemary, 29, Montgomery, AL.

X-Rays

I went to the chiropractor against my better judgment because my lower back was killing me. The chiropractor decided to take an x-ray to better see how to treat my pain. He asked if I might be pregnant, and I jokingly said that I didn't think so (although I thought I might be). When I found out I actually was pregnant, I looked back on that exam and had a terrible fear through my time. I had other fears too, that I may not be doing something right. My doctor and family said that it probably didn't affect her, and when I saw her perfect little body, I knew they were right.

Pamela, California.

I had an x-ray, for my shoulder, the same month I found out I was pregnant. When we found out about the baby, I was already six weeks and very fearful the baby might have suffered from the radiation. However, my doctor assured me that it more than likely didn't have an affect since the radiation isn't potent enough, and I was covered. Also, my shoulder isn't really near my abdomen.

Janey, Springville, UT.

Old Wives Tales

I'm certain that you will be and have been offered all kinds of advice and expertise from friends and relatives who have had children, so this section is dedicated to them. In each chapter, you will find a few old wives' tales, so maybe when you hear them, you'll smile and find someone with which to trade them.

A sure-fire way to get pregnant is to stand on your head after intercourse. Gravity will ensure your success.

If your morning sickness is severe, you'll have a girl.

If your mother had an easy pregnancy, you will too.

If your mother never lost weight after pregnancy, you won't be able to either.

Chapter Two

The Second Month II

"A baby is God's opinion that life should go on."
Carl Sandberg

You've made it through the first month, and it's on to month two. This month could be very different from or similar to the first month, and your body will change with every consecutive month. With most first pregnancies, you may not begin showing until five months, depending upon your body type. With my second pregnancy, I began feeling like a balloon at this point. I had already gained five pounds (in my breasts alone!), probably just from the excitement.

For many women, this month brings such side affects as food cravings or aversions, constipation, heartburn, and if you had morning sickness last month, it will probably continue on, even into the third month. That nasty film in my mouth lasted almost three months. Everything I ate and drank tasted dull, and I really didn't have an appetite. I still ate everything, but it didn't taste like it should have. I'd have to brush my teeth and gargle with mouthwash to get rid of the taste, and sometimes that would taste bad too.

In this chapter, the ladies cover many topics that occur in month one as well. This was the month of discovery for me with my first baby. You may have chosen to save your announcement until this month when you feel "out of the woods" or over the risk of losing the baby. At this point, too, I remember finally feeling comfortable with the idea of being pregnant, although the total reality wouldn't hit until month four and five when major re-shaping would occur!

Whatever your case, month two can be just as uneventful or exciting as month eight. I'll let these women tell you more:

Announcements

A close friend of mine had a miscarriage at about 10 weeks and hadn't told anyone she had been pregnant. When she told me that she had a miscarriage, I felt so bad for her. Because friends and I had heard the news of her pregnancy and miscarriage at the same time, it was harder for us to go through the mourning process with her. With her next pregnancy, she told her close friends and family immediately because she felt that if something did happen, she wanted to go through it with everyone supporting her. She had a healthy baby boy and never regretted her early disclosure.

April, 24. Utah.

Body Changes

At about eight to twelve weeks my nipples began to burn terribly. It felt like someone was holding a lighter and burning them! That went away at about 15 weeks.

Barbara, 22, Mackinaw, IL.

The most annoying thing about my second month of pregnancy was the break-outs I had. Around my jaw-line, I had the most irritating little, red bumps, and that's the only place they were. Some really hurt too, especially when I would try to pop them like you're not supposed to do. I tried dabbing alcohol on them, but it didn't work very well. The strange part was that the rest of my face was dry and flaky.

Maria, 24, New Mexico.

At about 10 weeks I started noticing that a burp would lead to vomiting. It was so gross. I would wake up starving in the middle of the night because I could hardly eat anything. The acids in my stomach were making me feel sick and full during the day. I tried over-the-counter antacids, digestive enzymes, anti-gas agents, eating slowly, no water with meals, chewing slowly, but nothing seemed to work. The incessant burping was the worst.

Gina, 31, Pennsylvania.

My gums were really soft and easy to bleed, and to make matters worse, the toothpaste made me want to puke. My dentist told me not to brush too hard, which causes the bleeding and receding gum lines. He also said to brush my teeth really well at night with toothpaste, and in the morning, brush with just water to avoid the vomiting. It worked well that way until I could stand the taste again.

Diane, Valrico, FL.

I had very low blood pressure during my first trimester. I felt breathless and woozie all the time. I almost blacked out every time I'd stand up a little too fast. I decided that since my job was flexible that I'd stay home and rest more until it all passed.

Loraine, 28, Deer Park, TX.

Cramps

I experienced terrible, painful abdominal cramps at around 12 weeks. I called my doctor about it scared that I was going to have a miscarriage, but she said it wasn't anything to worry about. She explained it as my abdominal muscles stretching to make room for my growing uterus. It didn't happen many times after, about 2 or 3, so I stopped worrying.

Cindy, 40, Montrose, CO.

At 8 weeks, I began feeling enormous pain in my lower abdomen when I coughed, which my doctor called Round Ligament Pain. He said it was caused by the stretching of the muscles of the tummy and all the organs moving to give room to the growing uterus. The pain mostly occurred when I was sitting or lying down. I found that when I had to cough, I either needed to stand up, or if I was in bed, it helped if I curled up in the fetal position.

Taylor, 22. Boston, MA.

Cravings and Aversions

My cravings began around 10 weeks and centered around Mexican food. I loved the cheese dip and the bean burrito deluxe with extra sour cream. I figured I was going to gain weight anyway, so I just began to eat everything I loved and never got to eat before my pregnancy. I'll leave out exactly how much weight I actually gained. Let's say I had to work hard at the gym later.

Maya, 30, Chicago.

I absolutely hated all food and drinks when I was about 6 weeks pregnant. It was all I could do to force myself to eat. It wasn't that I wasn't hungry because I was starving. I had only vomited a couple of times, but I felt awful all the time with gas and indigestion. The thought of food only made me feel ill at what it might do to me once I did eat. I thought the term 'food aversions' meant I would develop an aversion to SOME foods, not every form of sustenance. A craving would have been welcomed then.

Linda, Long Island.

I know it's not exactly a food, but I was very picky about toothpaste flavors. I had to choose a paste that had a mild taste to it. All the others would make me sick.

Laura, Jacksonville, FL.

I craved fair food. The fair came to our town about a half-mile down the road, and when I opened the window, I swore I could smell it. One night I talked my husband into going to the fair for dinner! We had everything, cotton candy, corn dogs, popcorn, pretzels, lemonade, pork chop sandwiches, anything void of nutritional value. It was wonderful!

April, 30, Augusta, GA.

Emotions

I was not prepared for all the ups and downs I experienced. I would go from resenting the fact that I was pregnant because it meant sacrificing my freedom to loving the fact that there was this little human that my husband and I created together growing inside me. I cried at the drop of a hat and never felt so out of control. I hated that part the most.

Katy, Ohio.

By my second doctor's appointment, I got to hear the baby's heartbeat, and it was wonderful. I went there feeling terribly exhausted and thought I was just working too much. The doctor told me I was anemic. Once I went home and started taking the iron, I perked right up. I felt so good that it was scary. I found a great iron supplement that didn't cause constipation, and I took it with vitamin c.

LaKayla, 20, Teaneck, NJ.

Morning Sickness

I was so nauseated that I really wanted to vomit thinking it would make me feel better. I couldn't even do that. I work full time and my colleagues commented on the different shades of green I had in my face. At the nine week mark, I went to see my doctor about this, and he prescribed Diclectin for my nausea. It took me at least a week before I noticed a difference. What a great drug! It was effective, but it didn't completely rid me of the nausea 'feeling.' I had to force myself to eat, and when I looked in the mirror, I thought I really looked pathetic.

Eleanor, 40. Montreal.

I had morning sickness terribly for almost 12 weeks before I tried wearing sea sickness bands on my wrists! My midwife recommended this trick. The bands were pretty cheap, and I would wear them all day. They significantly reduced the nausea, and they are drug free.

Lisa, 31, Cleveland, GA.

Pre-baby Journal

On suggestion I want to make to all Mother's-to-be is to write a letter (or a few throughout your pregnancy) to your unborn child. I wrote one the week we found out, one when I was about 5 months, and one right before he was born. I can look back on those now and clearly recall all the feelings I felt back then. Reading them still makes me teary. I also created a pre-baby book with ultrasound pictures, cards, pictures from baby showers, and then when he was born I continued it with pictures of my son, his hospital bracelets, etc.

Joanne C., Holts Summit, MO.

I am so happy that I kept writing in my journal during my pregnancy. I never realized how much fun it is to have the experience written down. I can share the entries about her with my little girl when she's grown, and I can compare experiences when I have another child. I may also want to look back and remember why I don't want to get pregnant again.

Marsha, Upland, CA.

Smells

Once while I was in our kitchen with an open window, I said "I think I just smelled a dog walk by outside." My husband thought I was nuts, but I was right! Also, my husband's breath bothered me at times, though it never did before.

Amber, Fort Worth, TX.

The aftertaste left in my mouth after I ate really bothered me, but not as much as my husband's breath!! After he would eat garlic, onions, or worse, smoked a cigar or cigarette, I would not go near him. It was terrible. And if he did smoke while I was in the same vicinity, say if he was outside or in the garage, I could smell it through the closed doors. I was miserable.

Melanie, Redding, CA.

My sense of smell was heightened so that my husband offered to go to the local pool to see if they had any nose plugs for sale. I could smell my son having a poop five minutes before he actually had it. I loathed going into the meat/ fish section of my grocery store.

Ella, 40. Montreal.

I could smell a cigarette a mile away, but the worst was people's cologne. I don't think people consider other's senses when they choose a type of cologne or how much to wear. I would have to back up from people because their cologne was just too much to handle.

Sarah, 49, Cheney, WA.

Old Wives Tales

If you crave meats and cheeses, you're having a boy.

If you don't satisfy your craving, no matter what it is, the baby will be born with it on his/ her nose.

If you crave sweets, you'll have a girl.

Chapter Three

The Third Month III

"If your baby is 'beautiful and perfect, never cries or fusses, sleeps on schedule and burps on demand, an angel all the time,' you're the grandma."

Theresa Bloomingdale

Around month three, my pants began to fit too snug around the waist, and I began showing some extra pudge, especially with baby number two. The nausea and nasty taste began to subside, but with that came new sometimes even stranger feelings. My pregnancy became more of a reality when I could actually see it. You know how we women can notice a new pound, much less five or more!

You may begin to feel more uncomfortable in your regular clothes and similarly uncomfortable in maternity clothes as well. This is a month of feeling "in between" as one mother-to-be calls it. I began wearing some maternity clothes this month with my second baby. I gained weight very fast, and the stretch waist pants were the best!

Some women just begin to realize and feel like they are actually pregnant in this month, with fears and dreams beginning to show up. I was always worried that the alcohol I drank before finding out I was pregnant had somehow hurt the baby. I would feel terrible if I had somehow done something to harm the fetus. I had weird dreams, wondered what my baby was going to look like, and worried if the baby would be normal. These fears can turn into unusual and strangely funny dreams.

Hormones are funny things, and during pregnancy they are going wild inside you, having parties and losing control, as they did with me. I found myself crying or angry or even happy all at once and at many different times during a single day. Don't feel bad if this is you too, and feel lucky if you don't experience similar emotions this soon or at all!

As your life begins to change and the pregnancy becomes more of a reality, becoming conscious of your body and baby's needs is essential. Getting into new patterns of healthy eating and exercising for me was very difficult. I wanted to eat everything in sight and felt too tired to go to the gym. I went anyway, though, and still gained an enormous amount of weight!!

If you are in a high-risk category, this month can bring relief or struggle. Many women can become diabetic during pregnancy, which is known as Gestational Diabetes. Other changes can occur and issues such as blood type, weight gain, and the baby's growth become magnified and closely monitored. Just remember, you've almost made it to the second trimester, and think positively! A positive attitude and mind will lower your stress level and relax your baby.

Here's more…

Body Changes

My hair drove me nuts from about 12 weeks to about the end of my pregnancy. I lost my natural curl. My hairdresser said that it was common, and that some women's hair, if it was straight, could get curly. Every hairstyle I tried worked for about a day and then flopped. I love how the hairdresser can style it beautifully, and when I get home, I can't make it do what the stylist did. My hairdresser suggested I grow it out while I was pregnant, and that's what I did. It got very long, and two weeks after delivery, I got a great cut.

Veronica, 28. Houston.

I had terrible trouble with headaches for about two weeks in my third month. I found that not getting enough rest was the main cause. I had to go to bed about an hour earlier than usual, and if I didn't, the next day I'd have a headache. I felt guilty about taking Tylenol, and my doctor said it was just hormones. I was told to drink lots of water to prevent dehydration and stay away from caffeine. I also found complaining about it helped me a lot!

Christy R. Tallahassee, FL.

Emotions

My wife was 14 weeks when I first heard the baby's heartbeat. I thought it was so cool. I realized that although she looked almost normal, that there was my baby growing in her belly. How cool.

James, 29, Baltimore, MD.

I kept a journal of my pregnancy, and at 20 weeks I was bummed all the time. I felt so "in between" because I hadn't felt the baby move or kick. I wasn't going to find out the sex for another 8 weeks. I was too big for regular clothes and not big enough for maternity clothes. It was an awkward period that literally drove me nuts, and I couldn't ask people how to deal with it because they all described their emotions differently.

Jamie, 33. Mississippi.

Fears

I had many fears about my pregnancy. At about three months, I began to feel the reality of the pregnancy, and I began to fear what I couldn't control. I was worried it wouldn't be normal, that he or she may be mentally retarded or deformed in some way. It sounds bad, and I tried to have a positive attitude. I just worried that the baby would be okay. This pregnancy has made me realize that I cannot control what is going to happen with my little one.

Jane, 27, Daytona, FL.

I developed a fear of toxoplasmosis during my pregnancy. I own a cat, an indoor cat, and he had even tested negative for toxoplasmosis. But I was still convinced I would get it and was terrified. I read all I could on the subject and even emailed people who researched it, but I was still scared. I had even stopped eating meat because I heard it lives in raw meat. I also had a fear that my baby wouldn't be normal or be mentally retarded. I feared deformity as well. I tried to have a positive attitude throughout my pregnancy, but the whole event made me realize just how much I cannot control what happens to my little angel in there.

Barbara P., Boston.

Gestational Diabetes

I had Gestational Diabetes with my second baby. I was so upset when I found out, but then I got educated…I read everything I could about it and went to a dietitian. I was able to control it through diet and checking my sugar level three times a day. My daughter weighed 8 pounds 5 ounces and was three weeks early. She had a slight low blood sugar level but was fine within a few hours. I do know people who have had to have shots without much discomfort.

Dee Dee, Hackensack, NJ.

I had Gestational Diabetes and was insulin dependent. The shots were no big deal. I used the ultra fine needles and could hardly feel it when I did it right. The first few tries were a bit painful. I was induced at 35 weeks due to the "aging" of the placenta. This is common in pregnancies that are insulin dependent and where the mom was insulin dependent in a previous pregnancy. I worked very hard to stay on my diet and always took my insulin. I only gained 11 pounds total for the pregnancy and my little "peanut" weighed in at only 4 pounds 13 ounces. Just be aware that if you do become insulin dependent, it is likely that your baby will spend at least two hours in NICU, so they can monitor his or her sugar levels. My son had to spend 24 hours in NICU because his were low.

Lucy, Franklin, TN.

I had Gestational Diabetes with my last pregnancy. It wasn't too bad and probably helped keep my weight under control. I had to take insulin shots, and that wasn't too bad either. I am a nurse and my husband a paramedic, so no big deal. My doctor induced me at 38 weeks. I found that taking a walk really helped get my sugar down if it got up. It seems like the pregnancy and diabetes will last forever, but it doesn't.

Jenna, 31, Warren, OH.

The worst part of my pregnancy was having Gestational Diabetes and having to give myself shots. I hate shots. Most of the time, my husband or mother would give them to me, unless I was alone, and then, well, I had to do it for my baby. That's the way I look at it. I don't have to have the shots anymore, thank goodness.

Kris, Yorba Linda, CA.

Maternity Clothes

Around 15 weeks, I began to feel very uncomfortable in my regular clothes. The really scary thing I heard was you usually don't fit into your normal clothes even after having the baby as your body takes a while to return to its pre-pregnancy shape. One friend of mine who suffered from quite bad post-natal depression said that one of the things that set her off was having to wear awful maternity clothes after having her baby. This was the reason I bought some stylish pieces like jumpers, baby-doll dresses and comfortable maternity jeans, so I won't feel completely terrible afterwards.

Nicole, 23. Washington DC.

I was wearing maternity clothes at 14 weeks, well more like a cute maternity t-shirt and regular elastic waist pants. These clothes made my life much more comfortable and people began saying, "Wow! Now you look pregnant!" The top rounded out my tummy, so I looked pregnant and not fat.

Leslie M. Colorado.

Around 16 weeks, I began needing larger clothes, and since I worked full time, I needed clothes I could wear to work as well. I found that many maternity stores in the malls sold expensive clothes, too expensive for my small budget. So, I found a consignment store that had great maternity clothes at reasonable prices. I didn't mind wearing something "second-hand" since I wasn't going to wear it for long, and for work, I needed more than just jeans and t-shirts.

Janet, 38. North Dakota.

Tests

When I was 16 weeks pregnant, I had a blood test called triple screen or Maternal Serum Screening. All pregnant women in Ontario are offered this test. It screens for down syndrome, spina bifida, and other birth defects. The results only tell you if your baby has a chance of having one of these defects, and if the chances are high, you are offered an amniocentesis. I felt that if I knew my child had one of these problems, that I would have an abortion, so I went through with the test. The test came back positive for Down syndrome, and I had a 1 in 100 chance that my baby would have the birth defect. I scheduled the amniocentesis. It was Christmastime, and the holiday was very stressful as we still had to wait for the results. I was surrounded by family who wanted to share in my pregnancy, but I couldn't share their joy. I would not allow myself to become attached to the baby until we had the results, and that was 3 weeks away. On New Year's Eve, my husband and I were lying on the floor with his hand on my stomach, and we felt the baby move! I looked at him with tears in my eyes, and we fell in love with the baby no matter what. By the time the amniocentesis results came back, I had felt a lot of movement; I was showing and glowing. The test results came back negative, and if I were ever to be pregnant again, I will skip the Triple screen test. It caused too much stress and the thought of a very difficult decision.

Sandra, 28. Ontario, Canada.

Weight Gain (or lack of)

I was 18 weeks pregnant with my third child when I had an ultrasound saying my baby was about 8 inches head to toe and weighed about 7 ounces. I remember feeling, 'Where is it? I'm not showing at all!' I had only gained 3 pounds, which was all in my chest, and I was eating 2200 calories a day. I always heard how lucky I was, but I didn't feel that way. I wanted to look pregnant, as weird as that might sound. I'm only 5'1" and normally 105 pounds, so I thought any little bit would make my tummy bulge, but I was still a size 3. I felt miserable, that is until I was about 8 months pregnant, and I couldn't wait to have the baby and get thin again.

Michelle, Kansas City.

I was 17 weeks and had only gained 1 pound according to my doctor. Except for my larger breasts, you really couldn't tell I was pregnant. My jeans had gotten uncomfortable, but that was about it for a while. My husband was more worried about it than I was. He was worried I wasn't eating enough and exercising too hard. I'm only 5'5" and 120 pounds normally, but my two sisters were already showing by this point. I ate more and exercised less than normally, but I didn't want to let myself go after I had worked so hard on my body.

    Grace, 25, New Orleans, LA.

At 15 weeks, I felt like a pig. I think just the thought of being pregnant meant I could eat anything I wanted. And the depressing part was I have a friend who just had a baby and is in perfect shape. Her delivery was a mere hour and a half for her second child, and she was up and about right after delivery. She said being in shape (health diet, exercise) made everything easier including losing the weight afterward.

    Maria, Lake Villa, IL.

Old Wives Tales

If you eat fish, you'll have a smart baby.

Eating strawberries will cause red birthmarks.

The number of a baby's heartbeats per minute can tell whether it's a boy or girl. If the number is high, it's a girl and low, it's a boy.

Chapter Four

The Fourth Month IV

A baby is…a rose with all its sweetest leaves yet folded.

Lord Byron

You are now entering the second trimester, which is considered the time when pregnancies are considered "out of the woods." Each month will now bring you closer and closer to the little bundle of joy at the end of this rainbow of experiences. And, as each day went by, I had another completely different mental picture of my baby. When I was pregnant with my son, I just 'knew' he would look like me, but the feeling was different with my little girl. It turned out she looked just like her dad.

This was the month when I began to get really warm, much warmer than usual, and I nearly froze my husband out of the house at times. I kept the thermostat at 68 degrees. The friends of mine who usually complained that it was too hot in our house now thought it was too cold.

This was also around the time I began noticing real changes in my body, size and function. Nothing seemed to work the same anymore, and embarrassing moments were right around every corner. I began to feel tired all the time, and I could only imagine what the next months would bring. I was really feeling pregnant.

Emotions are complicated things, really. Pregnant ones have been compared to roller coasters, elevators, balloons, volcanoes. Shall I go on? You and your significant other really have to keep a sense of humor. Mine were all of the above and at any given time at any given sequence. Just ask my husband! The water works sometimes came on while I was laughing!

Also, my sense of smell grew more acute. I began having trouble sleeping. I began worrying about the baby's room. Sex became an issue. The whole idea of wanting to become pregnant seemed more fun than how I really felt at this point. Phew! That's a lot to have going on at one time – and then pile on some housework...

Body Changes

I had really bad sciatica, which is pressure on the sciatic nerve that runs down the leg. Scatica can be caused by the softening of the ligaments and cartilage in the pelvis, which happens to make room for the baby and can throw your hip joints out of alignment. For me, this started around the 14th week of pregnancy and was wore in the middle trimester. I saw a chiropractor, but that didn't help. The pain in my hips was very bad when I would lie down, and some nights I had to sleep sitting upright in a chair. Nothing really worked for me, but the latest advice about sciatica is to keep exercising and walking.

Nora, Williamsville, NY.

I was thirsty all the time, terribly. I probably consumed 16 glasses of water a day, not including my 3 regular glasses of milk and any juice I might have had. All I could think about was drinking ice cold water. I even woke up in the middle of the night craving water, and then I had to go to the bathroom all the time!!

Grace, 28, Virginia.

I had a major case of the hiccups around my 16th week of pregnancy. I tried everything, and nothing would get rid of them. My husband made fun of me and said I sounded like a drunk on a three-day binge. He wasn't very supportive. My hiccups eventually went away, and then later on, my baby developed them. Needless to say, if it wasn't one thing, it was another.

Allison, 26, Detroit, MI.

At about 15 weeks pregnant, I began getting night sweats almost every night, and I never had them before in my life. I would go to bed and awaken in the middle of the night all hot and sweaty with the covers drenched. However, I got cold when I would take off the covers. It was so weird. I am normally cold-natured, so this was a new experience.

Patty, 31, New England.

I used to freeze in the middle of summer, being very cold-natured, but when I was pregnant, I could never cool down. I was hot all the time, including at night. I found that my deodorant didn't work the way it did before I was pregnant, and I had to re-apply it at least three times a day.

Nancy Y., New Cumberland, WV.

I began to have problems with my eyes around my fourth month. My contacts didn't seem to fit as well as they should have, and the prescription didn't seem to be quite right. My eyes itched and hurt all the time, and I went to wearing my glasses when it got too bad to handle. I had heard that a woman's eyes could change shape when you're pregnant, but I never expected it to happen to me.

Angie, 34. London.

Common Complications

Around four months we were told the baby had a single umbilical artery. They scheduled her for a tertiary scan to see the problems this might be causing. For a week we panicked thinking the worst, and it turned out they made a mistake. The baby was just in a bad position, and they couldn't see the umbilical cord properly. However, I did find out from people who had this happen to their babies, and none had problems anyway.

Lisa, Cumming, GA.

I had the worst flu I've ever had in my life at 18 weeks. I was miserable and stuck in bed for six days. I ran every day until I got pregnant then slowed down and eventually ended up sick. I hadn't been sick in three years.

Mitzi, Bay City, MI.

Around Christmas, I had a cold (19 weeks), and if I sneezed or coughed hard, I would have to strain to keep from squirting urine. I leak at least 2 times during the night. I thought I was going to have to start wearing Depends. I had a coughing fit at work once then wished I had wore a panty-liner. I thought bladder problems weren't supposed to happen until the eighth or ninth month, or until after the birth. I wonder if because I'm small everything was cramped and the baby was against my bladder.

Carolyn, Centralia, WA.

When people would assume that, because my husband and I are tall, that we will have an enormous baby, it infuriates me. In fact, my midwife says my baby will be average size and that the size of the baby of birth is not necessarily a reflection of the size of the mother. I was talking to a petite friend of mine one day who wanted to know what preparations I had made since stopping work. I told her I'd bought a Moses basket, and she said, " A Moses basket? There's no way your newborn will fit into it as I'm sure you're going to have a very big baby." I put her straight, but I was really annoyed by her comment.

Becky, San Jose, CA.

Around 23 weeks, I dropped a paper on the floor while sitting at my desk. I leaned over my belly to pick it up when the chair suddenly goes falling over me! I'm on the floor totally embarrassed. There were only 3 people watching me. Both of us were fine, except me psychologically. I had an even harder time getting up and dealing with all the bad jokes!

Sheri, Copperas Cove, TX.

Emotions

It was Christmas time when I was about four months. Between Hallmark commercials and my hormones, I had to keep tissues handy always. I bawled over everything sentimental. You should've seen me during the package openings. I received some baby things and just went crazy.

Angela, 29, Jersey City, NJ.

During my second pregnancy, I cried and cried and cried. I would get very quiet and introverted, which is not me. I heard songs and cried, watched TV and cried, and if my husband looked at me wrong or added a bit of sarcasm to his tone, I cried. It was terrible. Sometimes I would lie down and try to sleep just to try to make it go away. I thought I was supposed to be glowing and excited instead of depressed. It subsided at about four months and got worse again later.

Kris, Yorba Linda, CA.

For the first three months of my first pregnancy, I went along feeling pretty rotten all the time. Then, all of a sudden, I started feeling great! I thought, "Wow, this is great that I'm feeling so good so soon!" With my second baby, I didn't start feeling bad until the fourth month. Go figure.

Monika, 35, New Hyde Park, NY.

I was very lonely during my pregnancy. I worked with a bunch of men and knew no other pregnant women. We just moved to a new town with my husband's job, so I didn't really have anyone to talk to except him, and he didn't understand most of the time. My advice is to find some kind of support group and not go it alone.

Evelyn, 22, Leavenworth, KS.

Maternity Clothes

I am one person who hates nylons, and during my pregnancy, I could not find one comfortable pair of them. They were either too big or way too small, and the maternity nylons would slide down. Someone really needs to make a good, sturdy, and comfortable pair of nylons for pregnant women.

Wendy S., 29, Arvada, CO.

I finally had to shop for clothes around 24 weeks. I didn't like my shirts rising up over my butt. People were noticing I was pregnant anyway. I decided on soft, loose clothes because tight waists and some elastic waists bother me. Then, when I discovered I looked like a flowing tent, I went to a more business appearance for work.

Rebecca, Stevens Point, WI.

I tried about as long as I could before finally giving in to buying maternity clothes. I wanted to wear my regular clothes to finish out the summer before buying stuff I couldn't wear for but a month longer. They are so expensive. Also, I figured that eventually I was going to have to wear maternity clothes anyway. If I tried to go up a size, the legs didn't fit right or the shirt was too short in front.

Alyssa, Brooklyn, NY.

Baby's Room

We (I) decided to get started on the baby's room early. It didn't take me long to decide what I wanted. Since we didn't know what the sex was, I picked out something neutral, a combination of navy and white plaid (not gingham) and red material with tiny white polka dots. The theme was puppy dogs, so we sponge painted paw prints around the room. For the border near the ceiling, we stenciled red checkerboard. I was so excited about all the sewing and painting. And, I'm thankful for a mom who knows how to sew.

Corine, 42, Orlando, FL.

We had to totally gut our former spare bedroom and start again from the wall studs out, but I could already picture the finished room. We sponge painted the walls taupe with off-white over top and did a teddy-bear border around the middle of the room at the top of the crib. I got a honey-colored wood crib and teddy-bear sheets and bumper. I used a blind for the window and wanted an old-fashioned look all around.

Pam, Huntsville, AL.

Sex

Before I got pregnant and for the first three months of my pregnancy, my husband and I enjoyed a wonderful sex life. We had sex several times about every other day and I orgasmed without effort and often. When my belly started getting in the way, however, I lost the ability to orgasm. I felt sexier than ever, and my husband loved my pregnant body, but I missed the way we had had sex previously. I couldn't seem to concentrate on finding new ways and positions to make things better. Also, my husband is well endowed, and having less room made any penetration hurt. It got better after a while and back to normal later, but it was frustrating.

Nancy, Linden, NJ.

Not only was I having sexy dreams, my sex drive was through the roof (which is pretty unusual). I wanted it all the time. However, the dreams were pretty real. I kept having one about my chiropractor that seemed so real. I was really embarrassed when I went to my next appointment, and I really hoped I wasn't talking in my sleep!

Kim, Norton, MA.

My husband and I did not have sex once in the first trimester. Partly, I wasn't supposed to because of some spotting, but I also just didn't want to. In fact, there were times when I didn't even like kissing. Later, my sex drive began to wax and wane. Sometimes I thought I wanted to, then we would get started, and suddenly I didn't want to anymore. Other times, I am not in the mood, but my husband seduces me and I want to! It was frustrating for both of us. We were always worried about the baby too, like was he uncomfortable or could he feel anything.

Laura P. 33, Skokie, IL.

When I was pregnant with my son, I didn't want any sex at all. My poor husband. I still satisfied him in other ways, but even that was far and few between. It did create problems for us and a lot of tension. The most important thing is to discuss it with your partner and come up with an agreement you both can live with (even if you have to force yourself sometimes).

Jessica, Holts Summit, MO.

When I was pregnant, I was a sex maniac, really. I wanted my husband all the time, more than usual, which is normally a lot anyway. He loved it. He likes that we don't have to worry about getting pregnant and the fact that as I get bigger, we have to get creative.

Sally, Baton Rouge, LA.

Stretch Marks

I was so worried during my whole pregnancy that I would get stretch marks like my mothers. Hers were long and ugly, and they made any ounce of fat on her look like terrible cellulite. Well, I may be exaggerating, but I didn't want them. I used every cream there was on the market to prevent them. Around my fourth month, I met a man who told me, "You're not a real woman until you have the marks to prove it." I really took that to heart, especially when my husband told me he was right. Anyway, it made me feel better about the whole thing.

Judy, North Canton, OH.

I already have stretch marks from my first child, so with this last pregnancy, I didn't give it a second thought. I knew that if I did get more, I probably wouldn't notice them anyway. I have been told that stretch marks are hereditary, and I know my mother had them too. I guess they are more like war wounds or battle scars. I should be proud of them.

Marnie, North Creek, NY.

Old Wives Tales

If your hands are dry and chapped, it will be a boy.

If your belly gets hairy, you'll have a boy.

If the hair under your arms or on your legs grows quicker, or if you begin to find hair around your navel, it's a boy.

If your feet are colder than they were before pregnancy, you'll have a girl.

If your mother had stretch marks, you will get them too.

Chapter Five

The Fifth Month V

"A baby will make love stronger, days shorter, nights longer, bankroll smaller, home happier, clothes shabbier, the past forgotten, and the future worth living for."

Unknown

The fifth month is usually the time when we get to see our little angels for the first time; that is, if we want to. Some parents choose not to, preferring the surprise or having traditional reasons. But, there was a feeling I received seeing my child in the womb that was totally emotional and helped me connect to my baby. I have the sonogram pictures of both of my children taped inside their baby books. It was the five-month visit that showed a real baby inside my mammoth tummy!

Many parents are torn with deciding whether or not to find out the sex of the baby. I wanted to know with both pregnancies so I could decorate and be ready. Though, I have spoken to many couples whom, for various reasons, did not find out until the end. They decorated neutrally and bought very little until the day finally came. They found it fun to be surprised.

By this month, with my first I was very pregnant and wondering what I got myself into. With my second child, my breasts had already changed four bra sizes. I was spending all of my time in the lingerie store trying to find something comfortable in a size 40E.

Back pain was becoming a reality, and changes began occurring in my hair and skin. My hair never grew as fast as when I was pregnant, and I had beautiful nails. My skin on the other hand, I had broken out behind my arms and on my back with little bumps that didn't want to go away.

I was also writing at home during my pregnancy, and at this time I was working toward a deadline coming up soon for my book, *EMT Career Starter*, the second book after *Healthcare Career Starter*, which I also wrote while pregnant. I was getting bigger and less able to fit behind my computer. Reaching over my belly became a task as the months went on, but finding the energy and patience to sit for long lengths of time wasn't easy either. Besides, I had to go to the bathroom every 30 minutes!

What didn't help me was spending time with my neighbor and friend and her new baby. She also had twin three-year-olds, a boy and a girl. Her little baby was precious, and every time I looked at her, I saw my own little girl. That probably aggravated my situation more because I was all ready to deliver!!

The fifth month was like a teaser. For most, it's the middle ground between watching your figure slowly go away to waiting for the big day that will change your life forever. Patience is the key, something I have little of, and many other ladies found themselves in similar situations.

Back Pain

I discovered from a wonderful friend a way to help my back pain. Fill a brand new, men's over the calf tube sock with 2 pounds of uncooked rice. Then sew or tie off the top. Microwave the rice sock for 2 minutes. It smells great and it holds the heat for almost an hour. It also works better than heating pads that are supposed to be bad for pregnant women to use anyway.

Marsha, Grand Junction, CO.

For my terrible back pain, I would lay on my left side, stretch, do easy yoga positions, and sit with my spine straight. I also wore supportive shoes and walked regularly. It all helped me, depending on the severity.

Karen, Nashville, TN.

I wanted to tell how wonderful I felt since visiting a chiropractor. I had never seen one before this pregnancy, and I am convinced this is the way to go for mothers-to-be. I went initially because my lower back pain was unbearable. I was unable to stand straight at the sink and wash dishes for more than 10 minutes and sitting and sleeping were becoming impossible. My husband recommended the chiropractor. Since then, my back pain ease, and I've learned that expecting mothers who receive regular chiropractic care have shorter, less painful labors. Also, removing the stress from your nervous system will allow your baby to grow in a more healthy and safe environment.

Amy, 28, Bloomfield, MI.

Body Changes

I woke up at least 3 or 4 times a night to go to the bathroom. That started around 22 weeks and continued on until I delivered. The most irritating thing was never getting enough sleep at night especially when I had to work the next day.

Alice R, 30. Grand Rapids.

I had to get used to my new found breasts. I had to go bra shopping four times and each time would leave with amazement. I started out in a 36D and had to get a 40 because I'm short-waisted, and my belly made my bras uncomfortable. It was incredible. Then, not long after I was in a

40 DD. It took a little getting used to, especially the stares from men. How can they be so blatant? The sad thing is my butt grew just as much!
     Danielle, McKinney, TX.

     I began having ligament pain at about 20 weeks. Since no one warned me about this, I had no idea what the stabbing pain in my right side was. The pain was so intense at times and I felt a round hard place on my right side, which was sensitive to touch. One night the pain escalated to the point where I had to sleep sitting up, and this pain continued for a couple of nights. I got worried because the hard place was only on my right side, and I thought, what if it was a big cyst or something. I knew it was probably just due to stretching and the new weight of my belly, but my imagination was running wild. Finally, in the wee hours one morning I was moaning so much my husband decided to take me up the street to the hospital to be on the safe side. Well, the trip turned into an early hospital tour. Everyone was really sweet and explained about the stretched ligament and warned me about the discomfort level to come. Of course the pain disappeared shortly afterward, probably helped by some raspberry leaf tea bought in the health food store out of desperation.
     Carla, Bason, NY.

     At 21 weeks I passed my third kidney stone, and I could have done without that. The first two I passed were before I got pregnant. My doctor said if you're prone to stones at all that during your pregnancy's when they'll hit! This time, the pain was terrible. The doctors waited five days for me to pass the stone before they did anything. Finally, they went in, got the stone, and put in a stint so any future stones would just pass. The stint was sore and it hurt to urinate, but it was better than passing a stone. It wasn't fun and later on in my pregnancy, the stint was causing a problem and giving me intense pain. The doctor eventually put a tube in my back, so the kidney would drain into a bag instead of my bladder and any more stones that did form wouldn't cause blockage. Needless to say, my pregnancy wasn't pleasant.

Emma, 35, Metuchen, NJ.

Around month five, my hair started to frizz. It had always been coarse and dry, but my stick straight hair began to have frizz. I couldn't understand it.

Barbara P., Boston.

At about five months, I really began to show. All of a sudden people began to actually know I was pregnant. It was pretty cool because my friends were seeing a change in me. I loved the round belly and felt very comfortable in my maternity clothes. I wasn't sure I even wanted to get back to regular jeans after the luxury of the expandable waistlines.

Grace, Hilo, HI.

My breasts began leaking when I was only 5 months along. I didn't think that was supposed to happen until the ninth month, so it freaked me out. I heard it called "sympathy lactation," and it goes away.

Hannah, West Bloomfield, MI.

Braxton Hicks Contractions

The Braxton Hicks contractions really became a nuisance when I got to be about five months. I had a day where the contractions went from 9 am to 9 pm. Sometimes they were every 12 minutes then 8 minutes. They would stop for an hour, continue for a couple of more hours, and stop again for a while. I was really scared for a while, until I talked to my doctor. I thought I was in early labor.

Anne, Pocatello, ID.

I had lots of Braxton Hicks contractions during my pregnancy. Some were 3 minutes apart in my ninth month. I had to go to the hospital 3 times, but I wasn't dilated enough. The tightening would go all over my uterus and was sometimes painful.

Jeanie, 32, Van Nuys, CA.

Emotions

There were days when I felt good and then there were days and moments when I felt like I was absolutely losing my mind. That's when I would completely get stressed out. I felt like I had zero patience and would sometimes take it out on my husband. On the outside I tried not to let anyone know, but on the inside I felt like I would completely freak out at times for no reason. Taking walks helped, and I sure do miss a glass of my favorite Merlot at times.

Marty, Raleigh, NC.

I had two children 13 and 7, so when we found out I was pregnant, I cried for a week. Not out of disappointment, more from being scared and worried. We really hadn't planned for something like this. I was 20 weeks and had no clue, mostly because I was already overweight. It was shocking, but we got through it. That's when I finally realized what had been wrong with me the whole time.

Maggie, 39, St. Louis.

People at work kept asking me if I was all right. I hated it. But, there were just some days when I couldn't fake like I was the happy-go-lucky pregnant woman! I hate to complain at work because a "good, professional worker" always has a positive attitude about everything, blah, blah, blah.

Cary, Carrollton, GA.

Some days I would wake up and it would be all I could do to get out of bed. Other days I would bounce out of bed and rush around until I was exhausted. All I wished for during the last two trimesters was to have some balance. Instead I was spontaneous and unpredictable.

Sharon, Mason, NH.

Movement

I was about 21 weeks sitting on the couch watching television when, bam! I felt my tummy fall out from under me like I was on an elevator that stopped abruptly or at the top of a Ferris Wheel. My husband told me he was jealous, which I thought was nice. It is fun knowing no one can feel what you're feeling when the baby moves around. It's very intimate. I couldn't wait until she moved again.

Jackie L., Newport News, VA.

I felt so much movement from the baby. It sometimes felt like a football team in there. About a month after I first felt the movement, I found out there were definitely at least two players in there. We had twins!! One was quieter than the other, but they certainly let me know they both were there.

Samantha, Daytona, IA.

If my husband had been there, he would have thought I was nuts! Well, I had been lying in bed awake for about 20 minutes and hadn't felt any movement. So, I thought I'd wake the little one up. I took the clock radio and turned it onto a John Cougar song. I turned it way up and laid it on my belly. I was sitting there thinking how strange it must look. It didn't get the baby moving, but I figured maybe he'd end up liking good music.

Sylvia, Austin, TX.

Remedies

I drank eight glasses of water a day and was still constipated. My doctor told me to take fiber and recommended Metamucil, but I found better remedies in natural foods. I found I really love prunes! They are great cold. Also, dried apricots worked and coffee. I know coffee's not good while pregnant, so I didn't drink much, only about a half a cup. I also ate cereals like Golden Grahams and Raisin Bran for fiber.

Nadia, 25, Port Jefferson Station, NY.

I had a lot of yeast infections in from my fifth month on. I was told to use Monistat at half strength, and they would go away. I used lots of panty liners too to help combat.

Ruth, San Antonio, TX.

Revealing Gender

I paid for a second ultrasound out of my own pocket to find out the sex of the baby. The suspense was killing me, and the first ultrasound didn't show a thing. I don't like surprises, and I wanted to be able to decorate the baby's nursery, pick a name, buy baby clothes, and know who was growing inside of me before my child was born.

Blair, Madison, WI.

In both of my pregnancies, by about the seventh month, I was really eager to know the baby's sex. However, my husband didn't want to know and wanted me to respect his choice. Well, I have to admit it was fun and exciting when the doctor and nurses announced our little girl! So, for the second pregnancy, I decided to go through the suspense again, with our little boy!

Amber, Chalfont, PA.

I really wanted to know right away the sex of my baby, but we couldn't see her clear enough. She kept moving around making it difficult to tell for sure. I had been told that unless you actually saw a penis, that you really couldn't be sure what the sex was. I never knew for certain until I gave birth to my daughter.

Pam, Citris Heights, CA.

Rh blood type

I'm Rh negative and was with my first baby. At 20 weeks I had slight bleeding, was given the fetal cell test, which came back positive, and then given rho-gam. No antibodies were found. At my 28-week appointment, I was given the standard rho-gam, but my antibody test came back positive. I met with a perinatologist, and they did a level 2 ultrasound and everything looked fine. They seemed to think the positive 28-week test was a residual left from the week 20 rho-gam. They tested me again after four more weeks to see if the antibody level had dropped. It had. They monitored me very well throughout the whole pregnancy to make sure nothing went wrong. I had a shot before the baby was born to help with delivery and recovery of the baby.

Brenda, Chalfont, PA.

I am RH O negative and with both of my girls had the shots to prevent the battle of the blood types. My girls both turned out O positive. I didn't have any problems with the shots or any sort of after effects, and it, from my experience, isn't anything to worry about. This is a preventative measure for those with the RH factor. It's a good thing we're in the modern day now. When I was born in the 60's, they didn't have such a shot. My mother is RH negative, and they brought me on two months early. I was two pounds, 11 ounces, which at that time was pretty dangerous, and I died three times. With my sisters, they had to have blood transfusions immediately after birth.

Pam, 33, Citris Heights, CA.

Sonogram

At 21 weeks, we had our big day. I was a little nervous as was my husband. Both of us really wanted a boy, but we didn't care. The nurse had to do measurements first, and then we got to see. It was a boy! We saw him suck his thumb and roll over. It was the best experience, and we got it on film to enjoy later.

Tracy, 26. Kansas City.

My ultrasound went very well. We didn't want to know the sex, and baby cooperated by keeping her/his adorable little legs crossed the whole time. It was so incredible to see it waving its arms around looking like it was trying to punch me. The technician kept remarking on how much movement there was. The baby was in the breech position then. I was amazed at how thorough the technician was checking all of the bones in the arms and legs, checking the spine from every angle, measuring each section of the brain, checking the kidneys, bladder (full just like mommy!)

placenta, umbilical chord, everything. We got a beautiful video that was wonderful to watch later when my bladder was empty!

Elaine, Medford, NJ.

When we had our ultrasound at 22 weeks, everything looked good with the baby, and it was a wonderful experience. We found out that we were having a girl. I was very happy that the baby looked healthy, but I was kind of bummed that it was a girl. More so was my husband because he really wanted a boy. My husband and his father and grandfather are so close that I wanted a boy to be a part of what they share. I was really confused about these feelings at first, and it took some time for the idea of having a girl to set in with me and my husband. I didn't want to sound ungrateful, but we were a little upset having our hearts set on the hopes of having a boy.

Lisa, 24, Wilmington.

I was 22 weeks when we found out the baby was a boy. We saw him sucking on his hands, and he was very mobile. It was amazing watching him. His head was on my left side and his feet on the right. Maybe that's why most of my ligament pain was on my left side.

Beth, Auburn, MA.

We had our second ultra sound at five months. This was our first pregnancy and baby. It was amazing seeing our baby. The legs were pushing off the uterine wall. We could see the little spinal cord and its hand move the umbilical cord away. We saw the heart beating and little ears and fingers. The detail we were able to see was unbelievable and we have copies of all the photos.

Eileen, Mount Airy, MD.

Weight Gain

I had to inflict bodily harm to my husband at 23 weeks. We were watching television and this 7 month pregnant woman was showing her belly on some show. My husband said "Geez, you're bigger than she is." It was good that he doesn't bruise easily.

Tamara, Parsippany, NJ.

My whole life I have been obsessed with my weight, with losing and gaining it all back and losing again. I began enjoying not worrying about my weight. At 20 weeks I had only gained five pounds. The doctor was worried I wasn't gaining enough. I took care of that and had fun doing it.

Cathy, Williston, VT.

Here's a weight trick I heard about. Measure the top of your thighs. If the size stays around the same measurement throughout your pregnancy, you are gaining weight for the baby and not gaining body fat. The most helpful thing for me was a weight chart. I tried to weigh myself two times per week and believe you me I didn't deprive myself of anything; cookies were my downfall. But if I noticed weight gain, I tried to control my diet a bit better.

Rachael, Bronxville, NY.

Old Wives Tales

If your right breast is bigger, it will be a boy. If your left breast is bigger, it will be a girl.

It has been said that you shouldn't put your hands over your face or you will mark the baby's face.

Don't sit with your legs under your body or the umbilical cord could wrap around the baby.

If you look 'a little rough around the edges,' it must be a girl because girls steal their mother's looks.

Chapter Six

The Sixth Month VI

"People who say they sleep like a baby usually don't have one."

Leo J. Burke

By my sixth month, I began nesting. I didn't know I was nesting, though. I was constantly cleaning the house, discovering that the curtains hadn't been washed in ages and my son's room just happened to be too full of toys he wasn't playing with.

I was also out in the yard every day, even though my shorts weren't fitting well anymore, and I burned easily from the sun. I planted azaleas and worked with my roses daily. I loved to be outside; although the sun was hot and the days were long, I think it kept my mind off my size.

I went through a phase that summer, after having been a beach bunny all my life, where I wanted to tan but couldn't lie on my stomach. With my first child I was pregnant during the winter. That's easy enough, but this time it was the middle of the summer at the lake house, my husband and friends water-skiing, and bikinis everywhere. I was miserable in a good sort of way. I kept thinking someone needed to invent a chair with an adjustable center, but the sun is bad anyway, especially for pregnant skin, and there would be other summers.

I became more and more worried about the baby's room not being completed about this time. And, when I really get into the mood to do something, I do it and try to do my best. I was ready to put together a little girl's room. I stenciled roses around the bottom of the walls, which was not too much fun for someone so big. I had to lie in all different uncomfortable directions. My mother-in-law and I went shopping for furniture and searched everywhere until finally, at the end of a long hard day, we found the perfect bedding. It was beautiful. The room was filled with delicate, pink roses but still wouldn't be completely finished for another couple of months.

This is also the month when most women decide whether to take childbirth and breastfeeding classes and choose what type of classes to take. I didn't take any classes for either of my pregnancies, but I know women who swear by them. Also, many women want water births or home births and need the appropriate preparation.

The hardest part for me during my second pregnancy was around this time, my grandfather was diagnosed with a brain tumor. It was benign and the surgery went well, but I couldn't be there to support him or say good-bye if the case arose. I was miserable and 6 hours away. He was always like a father to me, and my hormones helped me suffer dearly over the fact that I might lose him. He was already 82 but in good health and came through the surgery like a champ, but I was still worried.

In any case, the sixth month means you're over the hump, and, if delivered, the baby has an excellent chance of surviving with today's technology. If you can survive the stress and strain of your new body this long, then you can be happy you're in the last stretch, the wonderful third trimester.

Anemia

When I took the test for gestational diabetes, the doctor found out I had anemia. I had to take iron supplements. I was always very tired and lazy. After I started taking the iron, I noticed a huge difference in my rate of motivation.

Emily, Rockford, IL.

I took iron supplements since my first OB appointment as a precaution. I was anemic several times in previous years (while not pregnant) and the main thing that I've always noticed was extreme fatigue. I noticed it in my first trimester when I was so tired. I could hardly get out of bed and just dragged all day long. No matter how much sleep I got, I was tired. I took my supplement with my evening meal because sometimes they were hard on my tummy.

Caroline, Danbury, CT

Body Changes

At 24 weeks I went for my regular prenatal visit, and for some reason I started measuring abnormally big. At 24 weeks I measured what I should have measured at 32 weeks. The next three visits I measured the same size, so at the 32 week appointment they were scared that the placenta wasn't functioning properly. Thankfully all was fine, and at the next visit, I measured at a normal 34 weeks. I have to say that it would have been comforting to know things like this do happen. Good prenatal care is essential.

Heather W., Canada.

By six months, the varicose veins on my legs were deep purple, and I had to wear very tight support hose, some my doctor gave me. They were terrible, and I hated it. I was never one who liked panty hose anyway. I couldn't understand why I had them so bad, I mean even on my arms in places and around my hips. I have been told it's hereditary, and I've realized it's no fun.

Lori, Bangor, ME.

I'll never forget this day as long as I live. My breasts had become really swollen by the time I was 27 weeks, almost to the point where I was miserable. But, if I was miserable, my husband took care of that when he looked at me, and with a grin said, "Got Milk?" All we could do was laugh.

Kelsey, 26, Burlington, VT.

High Risk Pregnancy

I had numerous problems during both of my last two pregnancies, such as placenta previa, ovarian cyst, anemia, intense low back pain, and during my last labor my daughter's cord was wrapped around her neck! My third pregnancy just recently was the same, starting with a persisting ovarian cyst on my left side again, anemia, and low back pain. The doctors just kept an eye on me, which is all they could do.

Beverly M., Canton, OH.

I just had turned 40 years old when I found out I was pregnant with my first. I had a relatively good pregnancy, no morning sickness or health concerns. But in my opinion, pregnancy is no fun at all. I was tired all the time, my feet swelled if I stood too long, my fingers swelled past my wedding band, and I could never get comfortable. My back hurt, and still does, my stomach hurt, my belly button hurt, food tasted and smelled bad, and I ate too much anyway. My husband was very sweet and supportive, but he told me I snored. Also, he's 34, so if I had had a girl, he would have planned my next pregnancy for a boy. I'm already 40, which is already high risk!

Gina, Duluth, GA.

I developed Prunitic Urticarial Plaques of Pregnancy, PUPP. It was a horrible rash all over my body that was incredibly itchy, red, scaly, hot, and uncomfortable. I had topical steroids, oral steroids, steroid shots and had tried every soak or cream known to man. The doctors decided to deliver my baby early scheduling me for an amniocentesis to check the lung functions and then inducing. Wow that was bad.

Lucille, Westbury, NY.

With two previous healthy vaginal delivers I found out that I had an abnormal AFP test and was diagnosed with placenta previa. After doing further reading on it, I learned that if the placenta doesn't move up before delivery, there is a chance I too could hemorrhage during a vaginal delivery. I was scared to death during the rest of my pregnancy. It was like a dark cloud that invaded my happy day. I was very careful, and the doctors did an early cesarean.

Lynn, Chestnut Hill, PA.

This was an extremely hard pregnancy, my fourth baby, and I developed Lymes disease. I was hospitalized for a long time and was very sick. The doctors tried to convince me to abort the baby because of possible side effects, but I couldn't do it. The other problem was that my last two deliveries, I nearly hemorrhaged to death. All seemed well with the baby, but I wondered the whole time if I should have had the abortion. Now we're glad I didn't!

Gayle, Greenwood, SC.

I had fibroids, one the size of an orange. I had to have a c-section and early delivery. There wasn't much room for the baby in there, and I was terrified throughout the pregnancy that I would lose the baby. But, the fibroids seemed to stop growing around six months, and the doctors were monitoring it steadily until the baby was born. I was very lucky.

Kara, Germantown, TN.

I had a tipped uterus and didn't really know until later on in the pregnancy. The doctor told me it would be no problem, until delivery. She said delivery would be more painful, and they would probably have to perform a c-section. She also said the uterus could tip back to normal. Well, the c-section went well at least.

Ellen, Glendale, AZ.

Movement

Some days the movement was just too much to handle. I couldn't seem to get comfortable and Jr. seemed to kick non-stop. I just wanted to shout "enough already!"

Sherri, Las Vegas.

I was 27 weeks when my husband finally felt the baby kick, and it seemed he wanted to feel it all the time. It was like he was thinking "Wow, that's our baby in there." Our doctor showed him how to find the baby's position by pushing on my tummy. That really got to him. He started talking to him, too.

Shelly R., Salem, OR.

My ribs were killing me by six months. They were always so sore and uncomfortable. The baby could be quiet with relatively quiet, gentle squirming and then all of a sudden start doing gymnastics. There were times I actually watched my bare belly convulsing all over the place as she squirmed around. At the end of a day, my insides felt like they were run over by a truck.

Ashley, Woodbury, MN.

Pre-term Labor

At 24 weeks, I experienced pre-term labor. I was having contractions and spotting, and there was bleeding in the placenta. I was put on complete bed-rest, and I was miserable and scared out of my mind. However, I managed to get a lot of stuff done that I had been putting off. I listened to a lot of books on tape, wrote memoirs for my baby (especially of the scary parts), caught up on letters to friends and family, organized photo albums, and I began addressing Christmas cards even though it was only July!

Martha, 35, Santa Fe, NM.

Sex

I was told by my family and friends that in the 2nd trimester (the honeymoon phase) I'd be wonderfully horny. Didn't happen. In fact, I cared little about sex and my poor husband. It made me sad because I knew sex was being put on the back burner and would be when the baby was born as well. My husband said the worst thing he did was get me pregnant. It just wasn't there for me, and when we did have sex, the experience just wasn't intense.

Sharon, Mason, NH.

When the worst was over, and I was in my second trimester, my libido pretty much went back to its pre-pregnancy state. My enjoyment level did increase somewhat too. I also felt more in love with my husband than ever before. Even when he was annoying, I thought he was cute. This was a huge improvement to the first trimester when I didn't want to be touched.

Donna, Fresno, CA.

God must certainly have a sense of humor. It seemed that while I was pregnant, the bigger I got, the bigger my sex drive became. How ironic is that? The only problem was that I felt so big that it really got difficult to enjoy the act, even when my husband claimed that he didn't mind how big I was. Then as time progressed, I wanted to have sex to promote labor!

Alice W., 30, Grand Rapids, MI.

Sleeping

I found that sleeping with one of those body length pillows helped me because I could rest my protruding tummy on it, wrap my arms around it, tuck it between my knees, even wedge my body against it facing down (kind of like sleeping on my tummy, which was my favorite position). It was easier to use one of them than arranging a bunch of pillows.

Beverly T., Stanford, CT.

Sleeping got to be such a major problem, that my husband elected to sleep on the couch most of the time, or he would sleep with me until I managed to kick him out of bed. My poor husband. I just told him to look at it like pay-back for all the times he wasn't going to understand me.

Julie, Dallas, TX.

I had to sleep with a ton of pillows by the time I was about six months along. I wasn't very big yet, but I was so used to sleeping on my stomach that sleeping on my side wasn't comfortable. I thought of getting a body pillow, but I wanted something smaller that I could adjust myself. I had three behind my head and back and one on each side of me, so if I rolled over, there would be a pillow there for my leg to rest upon. I had to buy more pillows and pillowcases to cover them. Then there was barely enough room for my husband to sleep!!!

Delia, 28, Louisiana

Since I was up 12 times a night to "go," I wasn't getting much sleep. I figured that when she came, that would turn into "nursing time," and I'd better get used to it.

Cheryl, 29, Ballwin, MS.

Twins

My first pregnancy was twins (no Clomid), the second was a singleton, and then we found out I was pregnant with twins again! I definitely had more nausea and fatigue with the twins, and my doctor made me stop working at five months as well. I was also a lot bigger than with my only non-twin, and I went through two girdles!

Tracey, Richmond, VA.

At 35 with two children ages 12 and 8, I found out I was pregnant with twins! What a shocker! My doctor said that because I am over 35 with a history of twins on my side of the family, that it was only a matter of time before twins came along. We were scared at first, but my doctor was very supportive and reassuring. I wasn't comfortable and used pillows and different positions. My maternity belt gave way around six months. Although, I did lose six pounds in the first trimester (before gaining 10 times that later).

Mary, Columbus, GA.

I think I threw up twice as much, was twice as tired, and was twice as crabby with my twins. I know one thing, that my back was twice as broken. But, then again, I was going to have double the fun later on!

Kristine, Redmond, WA.

At the six-week ultrasound, we saw one sac smaller than the other, and the embryos measured the same. My doctor said it could be nothing to worry about, but I was worried even more than I was already. I couldn't believe I had two babies in there, and the thought of losing one hurt me deeply. Well, at five months, all was in the clear. The doctors kept up with me, I had ultrasounds regularly, and two healthy girls. Wow.

Paula, 30, Lawrence, KS.

Old Wives Tales

Suspend a wedding ring or a needle from a piece of string, and hold it over your belly. If it swings side to side, it's a boy, and if it goes around in a circle, it's a girl.

Pee in a cup and sprinkle crystal Drano inside. If the liquid turns blue-green, you'll have a girl. If it turns muddy brown, you'll have a boy.

Hang your wedding ring from a strand of the father's hair over your belly. If the ring moves side to side, it'll be a girl. If it swings, it'll be a boy. Also, be sure to count the rotations that the ring makes to find out how many children you'll carry in your lifetime.

Add Clorox to your toilet water and urinate. If the water flows to the left, then it's a girl. If the water flows to the right, then it's a boy.

Chapter Seven

The Seventh Month VII

"Think of stretch marks as pregnancy service stripes."

Joyce Armor

By the time I reached my seventh month in both of my pregnancies, I was ready to deliver. The baby wasn't, but I certainly was. I was already counting the days until my due date and marking the calendar. It seemed that every entry in my journal had in it somewhere a sentence about how ready I actually was. I had dreams about my old, comfy jeans, good and bad, and I would go through my closet sadly, wishing for delivery. I was still attending the gym regularly but yearned for my old body.

I was stressed out by the thought of the past seven months. I had a short temper, and I think a little pre-partum depression. My son drove me crazy with his jumping and running around, and my husband couldn't do anything right. I found myself constantly reflecting on my family, how it would change with a new baby around, how lucky we were and how tired I was. I thought of the future mostly, about what she would look like and how both of my children would look and act when they got older. Would she be president? Would he be an artist? I still can't imagine the day that my son turns 18!! (What will I be?)

This was the month I began to think about choosing a pediatrician. Luckily, the best pediatrician in town just happened to have a child on my son's football team, the same one my husband coached. We had an in! In some cases, pediatricians only accept new patients once a year for a short amount of time because they become overwhelmed if they don't. Keep an eye and ear open for suggestions of good practitioners unless you're using your old pediatrician! Also, seek suggestions about childcare if neither of you is planning to stay home. It's never too late to look into good childcare, and most excellent care centers keep a waiting list!

Keeping busy each day seemed to keep the days from dragging by slower than the previous, and I was nesting more and more. It became increasingly harder to get a good night's sleep for lack of comfortable positions. I was also experiencing memory loss, especially when it came to my keys and sunglasses. One time, my husband found the toothpaste in the refrigerator! I didn't know what to say. Most of the time, he'd just tease me. By month seven, like most ladies describe, a sense of humor is extremely important.

Body Changes

I found that toward the end of my pregnancy I began to have problems processing and retaining information. I frequently experienced confusion and difficulty remembering things (short-term memory loss), and I used to tease my friends who had babies the year before about this. I teased them about losing brain cells to their children, and then it happened to me too!

Franlie, 37, Guelph, ON.

I was sweating practically through the whole winter! I even began showering twice a day just to keep reasonably clean. I couldn't wait for it all to be over. If that was what they meant by pregnant women glowing, I didn't want any part of it. Blech!

Stephanie, Greenwich, CT.

Childbirth Classes

I found the Bradley method to be the most attractive over the Lamaze method. Bradley focused on relaxation and visualization as opposed to the Lamaze method focused on breathing technique. It felt very woman centered and dedicated to a non-medicated birth. The husband or coach was very active and essential to the labor and delivery. I had talked to women who have done both Bradley and Lamaze and agree that Bradley is the best hands-down. Classes are taught by Bradley certified instructors and usually consist of 20 hours of training. There are also great books on the Bradley method if you can't attend classes.

Monica W., 32, Denver, CO.

I planned on breastfeeding but didn't have a La Leche League anywhere close to me. Although, they did assign a lactation consultant at the hospital (I was in Canada). I have a book that details, with real life pictures, the entire process. Breastfeeding sounded like a very challenging venture, and I didn't look forward to the pain of this very important aspect of motherhood.

Natalie, Boulder, CO.

Our birthing class was quite small (about eight couples) and was participation centered. We sat in a circle and were encouraged to have our say. We also broke into groups to do exercises on exploring hopes, fears, and dreams. This was a good icebreaker to making friends and to finding out who had similar ideas. The class focused on "active birth" and most of us were planning to have our babies in the birth center with minimal intervention if possible. Although, one woman said she was so terrified, she was leaning toward having an elective c-section.

Sue, San Diego, CA.

Our class was small with five couples total. We watched birthing tapes. One made labor look easy, and my husband said, "See, piece of cake." The second one wasn't so easy and made me want to punch him. I'm glad they showed both. We also learned breathing techniques and about what to expect from the hospital. In fact, half the question I was going to ask my OB/GYN on that next weeks' visit were answered that class before. We also learned about breastfeeding and breathing techniques.

Jenna, Lexington, KY.

Choosing Childcare

I began my search for daycare centers when I was six months pregnant. This may sound soon, but it wasn't soon enough. The waiting lists for the so-called "better" run center was up to two years long. My advice is to get on that waiting list of the daycare of your choice before you start planning your pregnancy.

Monica 29, Pennsylvania.

One of the most important things about picking a childcare center is to make sure the daycare follows all of HRS guidelines. For instance, HRS has a high teacher, low student ratio number, which ensures there are enough teachers for your child's needs. The daycare I worked for would have enough students to teachers in a classroom when parents of HRS would come to visit, but at any other time, they would have too many children in the class for the teacher to handle. This is their way of earning money.

Robin, Santa Monica, CA.

See if your state has an Info Line or Child Care Connections or some other agency that makes referrals. Child care providers (even home providers) have to be licensed here in Conneticut. I'm not sure elsewhere.

Check out the license for complaints on the daycare center. The things I looked for when visiting centers were: Does the place look clean? Is the food preparing and serving areas clean and diapering areas clean? Do workers wash their hands before and after preparing food and/or diapering? Look around for safety aspects, if the outlets and other such things are childproof, no sharp edges, dangerous toys, etc. Trust your instincts and ask lots of questions, everything from their sick policy to the discipline policy.

Stacey, Bridgeport, CT.

Check to see if there's a Child Care Info and Referral agency in your area. In Wisconsin, this non-profit organization is statewide. They can send you a while list of questions you should ask and you can also get a list of licensed and certified providers in your neighborhood/ city. They do ask for a donation to cover their costs, but it isn't mandatory. I found it very helpful. One thing you want to make sure is that it is okay for you to drop in any time. Make sure all medicines, other toxic substances, and sharp/ unsafe objects are up high. It's also important to me that the provider has first aid and CPR certification current. Ask about the classroom structure and daily activities/ lessons. You should feel 100% comfortable leaving your child there. I discovered that it's a scary reality that you can't trust those who are providing child care.

Nicole, Green Bay, WI.

Choosing a Pediatrician

Before I made an appointment to see a pediatrician, I made a list of questions to ask. Then I went on recommendations from family and friends and made appointments with two different doctors. I asked them about the different doctors in their practice and if I could pick which one I wanted to see. I also asked how soon after the baby was born do they see it (both said the next morning if it is born at night and same day if it is born during the day). I mostly wanted to know how they handled emergencies. I am a first time mom and know that every cough or fever can seem like the end of the world. They both had someone on call 24 hours a day and an answering service, which helped assuage my fears. Neither of the doctors I spoke to charged me for the visit, and they both gave me a lot of information about their practices and taking care of a newborn. They were very nice with pleasant personalities and took plenty of time with me to answer my questions. I had a hard time deciding.

Jenn, 22, New York State.

Circumcision

We did not have my son circumcised because it is not a part of our religion, and my husband is not circumcised. I recently read an article in a magazine that said it is not necessary to circumcise boys for hygienic reasons. After all is said and done, I think it is a very personal decision.

Roberta, Lawton, OK.

We had our son circumcised for several reasons. First, my husband insisted it be done. He is circumcised and remembers the teasing the uncircumcised males received in the high school locker room. Second, hygiene reasons were important. My husband personally knows several guys who were not circumcised, and later in life, they had the procedure because of infections. The surgery was much more painful, required many stitches, and took several months to heal.

Amanda, Birmingham, AL.

We didn't have our son circumcised because I did not want him to experience the stigma of being "intact" later in life. However, as I continued to research and found out how the procedure is performed, I found myself physically ill at the mere thought of putting my newborn though that. Additionally, if this is what he really wants, it can be done just as easily in later life. At least then, it will be his choice. My husband wanted it done "for hygienic reasons." I suggested that he speak with our midwife about fact vs. myth. I have found that many of the "ill-effects" talked about in horror stories are just myths. Furthermore, this procedure is so unnecessary that many insurance companies won't cover it.

Meghan, Knoxville, TN.

Movement

One night, around 28 weeks, I was lying in bed, and for about 10 minutes I had these little repetitious movements. They were in the same place every time and about four minutes apart. I tried pushing on my tummy, but he kept on doing whatever it was he was doing. My husband asked me what was wrong with him. I told him I thought he was having the hiccups but wasn't sure. This was our first baby, so we were constantly wondering what every little thing meant. Our son was very active. He would kick me very hard all day and night long. I was always wondering if he was ever going to sleep when he finally arrived. My husband and I are very hyper people in the first place, so I always assumed by his movements that the baby would be a bit too.

Maryanne, Sydney, Australia.

The first time I saw my belly move, it was very exciting. Sometimes I'd see a bulge sticking out and wonder if it was a foot or a hand. If I rubbed lightly, the baby would pull whichever body part it was away and move around. We'd always try to guess which body part was sticking out where then follow it to the rest of the body. My husband thought it was a great game.

Julia, Asheville, NC.

My little one did what I called barrel rolls. It was sometimes very uncomfortable and made me queasy. It was the weirdest feeling. I explain it like, when I was little, we would go visit my Grandparents on their farm, and to get there, my mom would drive up and down the gravel roads real fast to try and make our tummies drop. That was what it felt like. It was almost like I was falling, but it tickles and then made me sick to my stomach. I was always hoping the baby would run out of room sooner, so she couldn't do that anymore.

Fran, 23, Springfield, MA.

Memory Loss

I experienced major brain fade close to the end of my pregnancy. I am NOT a ditzy person (exactly the opposite), but I was a complete dweeb while pregnant. First, I lost my brand new cellular phone with no clue as to where it was. Then, I was walking at lunch and tripped and fell. Then my husband and I went to the grocery store, and we put the bags in the back of the car. I put a bag at my feet in the car, and that's exactly where it was the next morning when we finally found it. I about flipped since it had perishables in it that had to be tossed! Plus I would drop things, which really irritates me. I just felt stupid.

Audrey, Abilene, TX.

It's not really memory loss but a numb brain that I had. I smashed into a car that was parked in my own driveway. It belonged to one of my husband's friends that was over for dinner. The driveway is double-wide, and he was parked over to the far side. I totally saw the car and actually veered over toward it and ripped the back bumper off! I did even more damage to my own car! I couldn't believe it. I got to where I couldn't even back straight out of my own driveway anymore. The brainlessness was menacing. The car owner and my husband just teased me a whole lot. Physically I felt great, but mentally I felt retarded.

Tasha, Erie, PA.

I forgot where I was going all the time. I would get into the car, have a route in mind, and go the wrong way at least once a day. My mother asked me when my anniversary was, and I had to look on the calendar. A customer asked me how to spell my last name, and I had to look on my phone. The cashier at a store asked me for my phone number, and I just looked at my husband with a blank stare. I call it Gestation Brain. Who knew my baby would take all my brain cells too.

Charlotte, Gary, IN.

Pets

I was about seven months pregnant when I noticed my cat was acting funny. It was like she was on to my pregnancy. She began sleeping next to me, snuggling more when she used to sleep at the foot of the bed. She also wanted a lot more attention sitting on my lap more wanting to be petted or falling asleep. My family and friends (who don't have cats) were superstitious and kept telling me old wives' tales of babies around cats. They wanted me to get rid of her, but she is part of the family. I figured that unless she went psycho when we brought the baby home, we would all just adjust to one another.

LaShonda, Omaha, NE.

I have two cats, they were aware of my pregnancy big-time! Harry is 11 years old and can't stay off of my belly. If I would lie on the couch, she would get right on top of me. When I would move her off, she'd sit on my legs touching my belly. But, she never did get offended when the baby would kick her, which was all the time. Lance is 2 years old and started sleeping cuddled up beside me touching me in bed every night. He was always there when I'd wake up multiple times in the night. I had heard that through their sense of smell and your scent that they can sense the hormonal changes in our bodies.

Vanessa, 26, Fort Myers, FL.

Sex

My husband and I had terrible trouble having sex; it was a chore. No pain, just difficult to do. It was actually kink of funny. I just couldn't find a position that I would be comfortable with my oversized belly. We tried all kinds of positions but failed, and I endured discomfort. I wondered what would happen in the weeks ahead as I got bigger and decided we should just quit trying. I wasn't going to be pregnant forever.

Dori, Clearwater, FL.

Staying Home

I was terribly upset about not being able to stay home with my new baby. It just would have been impossible for me to do that due to the fact that I also have the benefits with my job. I am blessed to be a teacher. I would love to be home to take care of my child, but I think I would mess the mental stimulation, the kids, and the socializing that comes with being a teacher.

Carmen, Ann Arbor, MI.

I didn't want to put the baby in daycare at all. I was lucky to be in a situation that I could take the baby to work with me for as long as I needed to and/or work mostly out of my home. This job was the best decision I've made for myself. I stayed home with my first two and I know the feeling of being with them for every moment. This was a new experience for me because I would eventually have to leave him when he's much bigger. I have my mother-in-law to baby-sit, but it's still that sick feeling of being away from them. My best friend had to go back to work and was feeling that crunch. She pumped her breasts and continued to breast feed as often as possible. Another friend put her baby in daycare close to her office, so she goes over there every day at lunch to breast feed. I can't quit work, and I wish there were a better way for everyone.

Sonya, Mobile, AL.

Stretch Marks

My skin was great during my first and second pregnancy, that was the plus. The negative, however, were these horrendous, awful, terrible stretch marks, about ¼ inch wide and purplish black, all over my stomach. They went down my belly button too. They were horrible to look at, and all I could think about was plastic surgery.

Susan, Minnetonka, MN.

I had purple stretch marks on my hips, the tops of my legs, the underside of my belly and on my breasts, and I still had 6 more weeks of growing to go! I applied apricot kernel oil every night hoping they would just go away. All I could hope for was that they would fade after the pregnancy.

Candis, 22, Breckenridge, CO.

I have purple stretch marks from my belly button down to the tip-top of my legs. They go from hip to hip as well. When I wear my underwear, I don't have to see most of them, but I started getting them by my belly button. It really depressed me. I used a stretch mark cream with cocoa butter. It kept my skin smooth, and I hoped it will help them fade more. I figure, in the end you find it's all worth it.

Marybeth, Shelby, NC.

Weight Gain

My sister-in-law was also pregnant when I was and due not long before me. To hear everyone talk, she was the slimmest pregnant woman ever. She lost 12 pounds in her first trimester and had only gained 11 back from then on to six months. Her belly was big but cute. Everyone else said that she wouldn't get any bigger from then on. I, however, am pretty petite at 4' 11", and I gained a ton! My in-laws asked about my weight gain like it was a problem. I could still button my size 6 jeans at 4 months, but after that, I went crazy. I tried not to let it get to me, but with all the hormones, it was difficult. I was glad to have four pregnant friends to ride along with but was very sensitive to the comparisons.

Amber, Spokane, WA.

I've always been thin, but around 28 weeks, I began to feel fat and ugly. I never thought I would be saying those words. I had already gained 30 pounds at this doctor's appointment. I ate a lot and pretty much whatever I wanted. I felt gross and flabby and was so afraid it wouldn't go away. I kept thinking that after two more months I could go back to the gym, and that helped me make it through the last stretch. I didn't look too bad with lots of clothes on, but I hated the double chin.

May, Tyler, TX.

Old Wives Tales

If you have a lot of heartburn, your child will have hair at birth.

If you are extremely hungry, it means the baby is going through a growth spurt.

If you're carrying in front, its' a boy and wide, it's a girl.

Swimming in water over your navel could drown your baby.

If you lose your waist, you'll have a boy.

Chapter Eight

The Eighth Month

"A mother's role is to deliver children obstetrically once, and by car forever after."

P. DeVries

The eighth month can be the most trying time for any pregnant woman. You are so near the end of your pregnancy that you can taste it, but still so far away. Every ache, every uncomfortable sleeping, sitting, or standing position reminds you that you still have another month to go. At least that's how I felt.

Mostly, this was the month I was bored to death, in both pregnancies. I was so big, I couldn't move or fit anywhere. I kept thinking about writing but couldn't sit long enough to get anything written. I was uncomfortable and big. Two things I least like to be.

This may also be the time when reality, fear, and anxiety really begin to set in. You may begin to have what seem to be even crazier dreams. I had fears about going into labor. I thought about how lucky I was with the first labor being so easy and having an epidural. I heard stories about not getting to the hospital in time because the second baby comes faster and having to endure the pain. I learned about many different ways now available to birth babies from completely natural to water birth. But, being not very brave, I was nervous, excited, scared all in the same breath, praying for an epidural.

This may also be the time you begin having baby showers. I was given one by my family and a separate one by everyone else such as friends, colleagues and family friends. At the shower given by my family, they passed around a pad for everyone to write down a name for the baby. There were many cute names as well as the one I had already picked. I had guessed some people liked the name I picked. The ladies in this chapter have some great shower stories and there are some great party ideas in the back of the book.

Choosing a name for your baby can be a hectic experience, especially if you and your husband or other family members don't agree with the names you've chosen. My husband literally didn't want anything to do with choosing a name, but he would turn his nose up at every name I picked. My son liked every name I read aloud. No one was any help.

So, like many other women, you too are in the month where every night before you go to bed and every morning before you muster enough energy to get out of bed, you pray that your joyous days being pregnant will end soon! Don't get me wrong; I did enjoy both pregnancies. Many women love being pregnant. I just wouldn't want to be pregnant all the time!

Anxiety

Before my wife got pregnant with our first child, she miscarried once and after she had told our friends and relatives. It was very traumatic and I remember with the second the emotional roller coaster that we went through every time she felt pain of any kind. I think it's absolutely normal to worry, especially in the first critical trimester. It also took us about two years and some fertility drugs before she got pregnant, so that adds to the stress when you think something might be going wrong. It's okay to worry and by all means contact your doctor when you feel it necessary. But, enjoy it. It's the most rewarding thing you'll ever experience. We waited until our early 30's to have children, and it's been well worth the wait. It's hard to imagine now what life was like before the kids. There's nothing like holding that newborn after delivery. It'll be worth all the worry and stress that you feel now!

Robert, Des Moines, IO.

I wondered if I was going to be a good mother and doing the right things. It is tough for a first-timer, and people compare what you do to what they did or do. I had questions like, what if something goes wrong, how will I know what to do? My one older brother put it this way, "If you like roller coasters, hang on because this is going to be the wildest ride you've ever experienced. You will go from scared to tired to excited to scared again and at the end of it all, you will look down and see your child and know that no matter what else happens this is the moment in your life when everything makes sense. You will love that child and never be able to imagine what your like would have been like without him or her."

Kyra, Syracuse, NY.

I felt feelings of being unprepared, but I was tired of carrying the baby. Friends of mine had already given birth, and I was huge and tired. I was a college student and would deliver mid-semester. I had insomnia, swelling in my legs, I couldn't tie my shoes. And someone tell me why when I wasn't looking, my thighs got humongous. It just wasn't any fun there at the end, and I was totally miserable thinking about losing weight.

Charlotte, Gary, IN.

Body Changes

Fearful that I may go into labor, at 7 months I decided to trim my pubic hair, but I couldn't see it. So, I asked my husband to do it for me. We were laughing so hard that I lost control of myself and peed all over him and the floor!! I was so embarrassed, and my bladder control problem only seemed to get worse!

Barbara P., Boston.

It was terrible! I was eight months pregnant and still a 36B!!! I finally got to wear a bra extender at about 24 weeks, but I just never grew more than that. I thought it just wasn't fair. This was my one shot at big breasts, and I had terrible anxiety about breast feeding.

Rachael, 21, Alabama.

I had terrible hemorrhoids that were the size and color of ripe purple plums. There were at least three of them. I discovered a solution. Cut up bed pads, soak them in water, roll them into a large cigar shape, freeze them and apply them wrapped in a cloth. This was the best solution for me when hemorrhoid creams did nothing to dispel the pain and discomfort. The next problem was the inability (or unwillingness) to have a bowel movement and that resulting associated discomfort!

Franlie, 37, Guelph, ON.

Childbirth Classes

I decided to take breast feeding classes after a lot of thought on the subject of breast feeding. I wasn't sure if I wanted to do it, but I thought if I did choose to breast feed, then I might want to know how. The classes discussed problems women have such as infections, soreness, and latching problems, but the class also went over the positive aspects like the close bonding and the mother's milk strengthening the baby's immune system. The classes showed the pros and cons and helped my decision later.

Charlotte, Gary, IN.

The breastfeeding class slightly overwhelmed me. I didn't think breastfeeding would be that much work or that there could be so many complications involved. I had anxiety after the classes, and then I began to realize that women have been breastfeeding since the dawn of time. However, after my husband went to the class, I don't think he'll ever look at my breasts the same way again.

Leslie R., Eugene, OR.

I didn't take Lamaze but the Bradley Method. There were 12 classes, and we spent 10 minutes on "relaxation" techniques in each class. We were asked to practice at home what we learned from each class. I learned that depending on the individual, massage could either be great or really irritating. I found it really irritating. The classes also emphasized exercises such as Kegel exercises and pelvic tilts, nutrition, the normalcy of childbirth, and natural drug free birth. They also introduced topics such as the possible dangers of ultrasound, circumcision, unnecessary medical interventions and how they can do more harm than good. I enjoyed the different viewpoint from the standard.

Stacy W., 29, Connectuit.

I enjoyed the Lamaze classes I took. The more I attended the classes, the more aware I became of what was going to happen to me during labor. I was very nervous during the first class, but as we went along and discussed the birth process and practiced relaxation techniques, my anxiety was eased. My husband got a better idea of what was going to happen and how to help me as well; although, he wasn't so sure about the delivery after watching the birthing video. Also, they were held at the hospital I was going to deliver in, so I had the chance to become familiar with the facility.

Regina, Flint, MI.

I was distressed from my prenatal classes. They would talk about labor and delivery and contractions. I understood what happens during delivery, and I knew that labor was the work leading up to the delivery. But, since I had never had a baby before, I didn't know what a contraction was! What would it feel like? Would it hurt? This is what scared me the most. I talked to friends to find out, and they said it was like having menstrual cramps. I had never had menstrual cramps before, so I was back to square one. When I did finally go into labor, I experienced back labor and the most painful back pain I had ever had. It never felt like anyone described, until after I had the epidural, which was described as heaven.

Deanne F., Goderich.

Dreams

I had this dream that I was trying to breast feed my little boy, and when I looked down, he had a beak. When I looked again, he had lips and then a beak again. I woke up a little worried.

Tonya, 33, Wilmington, DE

We were in the hospital, and I had already given birth. My husband and I took a walk to see the babies. When the nurse pointed at our baby, I stood there in shock. All of the babies in the nursery were beautiful, except mine. It was hideous.

Marsha, Anaheim, CA.

I woke up one night at about my eighth month with night sweats. I had dreamt that my husband did not make it to the hospital on time for my delivery.

Janet, Clarksville, TN.

My dream was about getting home and realizing we had forgotten the baby at the hospital.

Sandra, Elizabethtown, PA.

I dreamt I gave birth to a 40 pound male baby with long hair and a mustache. I can only imagine what it was that I was eating that night!!

Taylor, 23, Atlanta, GA.

I had a dream that my water broke, and because of the possibility of a prolapsed cord, we had to get to the hospital right away. I was getting dressed and yelling at my husband to hurry up, we had to go, and he just lay in the bed saying, "okay, okay, give my 15 more minutes." In the dream, I got dressed and told him, "Well, I have to go!" and he said, "Okay, I'll be there in a minute." So, I drove to the hospital alone, and had my c-section alone with my husband still at home asleep! The terrifying thing was that was just like him to do that. I tried to wake him about a year ago when I thought someone broke into the house, and he was unable to get his butt out of the bed! That's when we got a dog. I told him about the dream, and he insisted that he would wake up. It ended up that he didn't have to.

Ansley, Brevard, FL.

Emotions

I experienced extreme hormones around my eighth month. I hadn't had any real mood swings since I was in my fifth or sixth month, but as this time, I started crying and couldn't stop. The worst part was that it all started because I didn't have anything to wear. All my maternity clothes were for the summer. My husband didn't know what to do and ended up picking an outfit for me. I think that I just wanted the baby to be born already. I felt huge, and I could barely move. I just got tired of all the attention and awkwardness.

Delta, Charleston, SC.

All I wanted to do throughout my whole last pregnancy was cry, and cry I did. Usually I'm not someone who cries so easily, so this was very hard on me. I am also very happy with a wonderful husband, great kids, and a much-wanted pregnancy. But, I couldn't stand it when I'd start crying, and I don't remember doing it with my last pregnancies.

Connie, Waco, TX.

I remember sitting in church one Sunday, and for about ten minutes, I kept crying and couldn't stop! I didn't know why either, and my husband couldn't figure me out. I was so embarrassed, which probably led to more crying. I don't live close to my mom, and going to church always makes me feel homesick, and I was probably feeling guilty about not going to church as much as I should!

Cassie, Huntsville, AL.

Hospital Tour

We toured two different hospitals where our doctor works. The first one was nice, big rooms, nothing out of the ordinary from the standard hospital room, but the size and the extra baby bed. The second one was all redone with homey type rooms with a big bathroom and shower, hardwood floors, etc. I chose the first one for a couple of reasons. The staff didn't seem as busy, and everything was on one floor such as, the birthing room, postpartum, surgery (if need be). The other hospital was fancier, but I would have had to switch floors after birth. Also, they only had three rooms finished, and I could've gotten a really old, teeny room if the others were taken.

Bridgett, Jackson, MS.

Movement

When I would tickle my belly, the baby would respond by thumping and kicking. It happened every time and really freaked my husband out. When I was pregnant with my son, I would tap the right lower side of my abdomen with a pen, and he would do a little jiggle across the center of my belly. I always wondered if they liked that interaction or did it annoy them? Is it cruel for me to have done this? I just loved watching the baby move.

Tammy, Vancouver.

My husband couldn't believe how strong the kicks were when I would lay down to go to sleep. Since I read that the baby is lulled to sleep when the mother moves rhythmically, I would sometimes get up and walk around for five minutes or so. When I felt lazier, I just laid in bed and rocked back and forth for a bit. It usually settled the baby down, at least for a while.

Loretta, Memphis, TN.

Naming Baby

Choosing a name for our baby was nerve-racking. My husband was really getting on my nerves. We couldn't agree on any names, boy or girl. He hated everything I liked and I hated everything he and everyone else liked. So, we made a list of all the names we liked, separately, and compared them hoping there would be one common name between them. That actually worked for both the boy and girl name.

Marsalla, New Mexico.

Our baby was lucky he got named at all! I almost just kept calling him "little boy." We had found out we were having a boy, and from that moment, my husband wanted him to have the family name Richard making him the second. I didn't want that. I wanted a name that wasn't as common and a name someone couldn't shorten or make a nick-name from. Talk about a subject that almost caused a divorce!!

Louise, 30, Portland, OR.

Nesting

Around 33 weeks I began noticing that I was doing some serious nesting. One Sunday while we were sleeping in, my husband noticed a tiny little stain on the bathroom wall that we had never noticed before. The next thing I knew we were pulling wallpaper off the walls and picking out paint colors. I think he was nesting also. We changed every room in the house and were thinking about the garage when the baby came!

Alicia, Doylestown, PA.

One day, while I was on my hands and knees scrubbing the kitchen floor, my husband came home early from work. He couldn't believe what I was doing, which made me happy, and told me to stop and let him finish. I almost passed out from shock, but he did finish. What a husband! I never thought it could be that good. It was short lived, since he never did that after the pregnancy, but I really felt loved that day.

Mindy, Reston, VA.

We have a really huge back yard, and although I do love to plant and garden, I have never done as much as when I was recently pregnant. I planted more bulbs, shrubs and azaleas than I must have noticed because the back yard was absolutely beautiful when Spring came. Flowers were popping up everywhere that I had forgotten about. My husband and mother called it nesting.

Jasmine, Clarksville, TN.

My sister told me I was nesting when I described wanting to knock out a wall and make the nursery larger. She said that's when you begin feeling like you need to prepare for your new addition to the family. I guess subconsciously I must have been thinking the Queen was coming because I really wanted to knock that wall out. My husband just said, "No way!" and just left it at that. He's not any fun.

Janet, Santa Ana, CA.

Open Nursery

I guess I was about eight months pregnant when my husband and I finally finished the nursery. We worked really hard on it and had a great time doing it all. However we wouldn't let anyone see it prior to it being finished, so it would be a big surprise to everyone. We finished washing all the clothes and bedding and had the room finished to the detail. Then we had an "Open Nursery" with my husband's parents and my parents, as well as friends and neighbors. I served cookies and milk to go along with the kid theme. We got the stroller and car seat out and practiced with a doll in them. It was really fun.

Brenda, North Adams, MA.

Showers

My mom threw me a huge shower, which was supposed to be a surprise, but I knew about it and just acted surprised. The women of the family were invited, and everything was beautiful. I never dreamed I would receive so many great gifts, and I got a lot of necessities. We also played a great shower game I would recommend to anyone called "Name the baby food." Everyone was supposed to guess what was in the jars and write it down on paper. The winner received a basket of candy and gifts. It was so much fun because only the mothers of the group had even a clue about what was in the jars!!

Louise, 25, Owings Mills, MD.

When my husband and I found out we were having a boy, he was excited. His best friend and he concocted this idea that if I was having a shower, then they should have one too. Most men I know wouldn't want a shower thrown for them, but not my husband. So, a bunch of his work buddies and close friends got together and threw a party for him to give him baby gifts. He came home with a baby work-bench and tools, a baby football, a baby baseball and bat, and other such gifts. I thought it was just an excuse to get together to drink beer and smoke cigars, but it turned out to be a hilarious idea!

Valerie, 35, San Francisco.

During my shower, my father and husband showed up with a delivery. They unloaded a dresser and brought it into the front living room of the house. It had a note on it that said, "To baby, love grandma and grandpa." The dresser was beautiful. Later, after everyone had left the shower, I discovered that in each of the little drawers my mother had placed a tiny gift. I spent hours after the shower unwrapping each one and crying.

Sandy, Harlan, IA.

At my shower, my friends played this great game that was so much fun. Each person was given a ball of yarn to cut a piece. They were to guess how big around they thought I was. The winner received a gift basket. It was really depressing when the yarn didn't fit around me, but it, ironically, was great when the yarn wrapped around me twice!! The winner was the closest fit because no one got it right!!

Sheila, Rodchester, MN.

I was having trouble trying to figure out how to get everyone I wanted at the shower my mother was throwing me at home when my best friend at work solved the problem for me. She announced to me surprisingly that she was going to throw a shower for me at work. I work at a plant that is open 24 hours. The shower was at 5:00, so both friends from the day and night shifts could come by the break room. It made me so happy because I have a lot of friends at work.

Jessie, Whitby, ON.

I went to a shower while I was pregnant and played a new game that I hadn't heard of. You use four sugar cubes and write B's, A's, and Y's on all sides, like dice. Three or four plates are going around. Roll the dice and pass the plate on. If you spell B-A-B-Y with the 'dice," grab a prize (there were two circulating). The plates keep getting passed for five minutes. Each time a person rolls B-A-B-Y, they grab a gift from whoever has one. At the end of five minutes, whoever has the gifts keeps them. It was a really fun game.

Brie, Dedham, MA.

I had a great time at my shower. My sisters decorated with a Mother Goose theme. They actually made little cows, moons and dishes out of color cardboard, tossed glitter all over them and strung them on the new "icicle" type of twinkling lights. The light cords all bunched up, so they tied kitchen spoons to the bottoms of the cords and strung these all over the living room. We all had glitter in our hair and on our clothes. They had three cakes, a moon, a star and a cow. They bought white and black chocolate in the shapes of stars, suns and moons and wrapped them in electric blue cellophane and typed out nursery rhymes on each little package for take-home treats. They must have planned the shower for months!! I received a lot of "abnormal" shower gifts, not the things you usually get like blankets, towels. I got big items like a playpen, a high chair, three or four outfits per box and 100 boxes. I didn't know the sex, so there were so many cute little girl/boy outfits. All I had bought was white stuff.

Ally, Bloomington, IN.

Weight Gain

I believe I lost my feet at about 33 weeks. All I saw was belly, or baby. I sure couldn't wait to have a waist again. I would have loved to be able to put on a pair of jeans with buttons and a zipper. It kind of makes me wonder where else the baby could go, I mean I felt I was running out of room. And, I had more weeks to go still.

Chris, Cincinnati, ON.

My friends all kid me because I've had four children and look like I've had none. I guess it's genetics or working out. With each child, I seemed to gain more than before. With my third, I got to 200 pounds and swore that wouldn't happen again (I knew we wanted another child). But, my fourth pregnancy took me to 220 pounds. I'm not having any more children, but not because of the weight gain. Gaining it was fun, but when the pregnancy was over, I was ready to get back to normal. I just couldn't believe I was actually over 200 pounds! I'm normally 5'10" and about 135.

Heidi, Potomac, MD.

Old Wives Tales

Don't dance while you're pregnant or you'll have your baby early.

If you get red highlights in your hair, you'll have a girl.

A big belly means a big baby.

Don't raise your arms over your head or the umbilical cord could wrap around baby's neck.

If you are carrying high, it's a girl. If you are carrying low, it's a boy.

Chapter Nine

The Ninth Month

"There was never a child so lovely but his mother was glad to get him asleep."
Ralph Waldo Emerson

If one minute you're exhausted and the next you're busy mopping the floor, wondering where this new found energy came from, then this is the tell-tale sign that you've made it to the home stretch, the ninth, glorious month. It won't be long now, if you weren't early already, until you have a brand new bundle of love and joy in your arms! Although, that thought is at most times hard to believe.

I worried about everything in my ninth month, like my water breaking in the supermarket, and hoped each day that the contractions would start. I remember going to my last doctor's appointment and begging him to induce labor right then! All I wanted was to be able to sleep on my stomach again. My clothes were tight, the baby's feet stuck in my ribs, my feet were swollen, and I felt like a stuck pig. Again, patience is not my strong suit. The new responsibility was right around the corner too, and I was curious about how my husband would fare with changing diapers.

Dragging my son and his friends everywhere during the beginning summer months wasn't much fun either. We were in one playground or another, at the movies, the mall, and friends' houses. I was so tired by the end of the day from just being pregnant that having a 6 year-old made it that much more tiring, and I only had more joy to look forward to since they were getting out of school at the same time I would deliver.

Make sure to pack your bag and have it ready by the door to grab at any moment's notice. There are some great ideas here. Have your chosen babysitter ready, if you need one for older children, and cook some meals to put in the freezer for later. Then get prepared for your ride to the end. Of course, labor should not be considered the end of anything, but since this book is about pregnancy only, we'll look at the pregnancy's end and save labor stories for another book.

There's something special and reminiscent about month nine once you've gotten here. It gave me a feeling of success that I made it through. And, the stories in this chapter are just as fun, if not funnier, as the past eight chapters have been. But like reading the pages of a journal, the experiences are best looked back on. Has it been fun for you? Or a rough roller-coaster ride filled with bumps and turns. Every pregnancy is different. I hope at least that has been proven within these pages.

Advice

I was finally glad to be away from work when I left in my ninth month. It was terrible having to work around all the self-made OB/GYNs there. The ones who swear you've dropped every day or who give you a panicked look when you tell them you still have x weeks to go. The ones who argue amongst themselves about when your baby is coming ("No it's going to be the 18th -that's when my cousin had her baby"). The ones who make comments all day long about how tired you look but don't do a thing when they see you hauling boxes around. And men, men are the worst. They say I look like I'm going to pop, and how can I go another day because I am so big! I mean talk about insensitive!

Marissa, Newburgh, NY.

I worked with a guy whose wife had recently had a baby. Whenever he would see me, he would take the opportunity to point out what I should and shouldn't be eating. It drove me nuts after a while. I had a small chocolate cookie at an office party, and he proceeded to tell me how bad chocolate is for me and that I can't have after the baby's born if I nurse. My response was, " Watch me!" I used to catch other people at work watching what I eat. They would point it out if I had more to eat than I used to. If I didn't eat enough to satisfy them, they'd point it out. I wanted to eat in the closet! Maybe the old days weren't so bad when women went into hiding during pregnancy. At least then I'd have gotten some peace and quiet.

    Madison, Raleigh, NC.

At work, any time I was carrying a mug, they would ask, " Does your doctor say it's okay to drink coffee?" I'd say, "it's not coffee but plain decaf tea." And every time I was seen with food, whoever passed by would take a close look at it to give their approval. I didn't like the comments. One guy (with a loud mouth) said to me, "Nancy, you're filling out! Ha-Ha-Ha." I just glared at him. I hated it when men in particular, would try to pat my belly. My friend's boyfriend was always telling me to come over to him, so he could pat my belly. It made me want to punch him.

    Glen Allen, VA.

A perfect stranger who I had two conversations with on the telephone came over to my desk to pick up a floppy disk from me. She was in a big rush to get this information on disk. Anyway, as soon as she saw that I was pregnant, she asked if I was going to breast feed. Then she went into a 15 minute lecture about the benefits of breast feeding, how long you should breast feed, etc. She went back to the caveman and through the horse and buggy days, and on and on. All the while I'm thinking, "What about that big rush you were in?" and wondering what I wanted from the snack machine.

Alex, Muncie, IN.

Don't you just LOVE the remarks such as, "You're due when? But you're so big!" and "Are you sure you're not having twins?" What about the hellos said to your tummy and not your face, and (this is a real doozie for me) the advice on what you are eating, drinking, wearing, saying, and thinking?! When did society suddenly get so intrusive over something that is really so personal to a woman? All this "interference" (for want of a better term) is very intrusive. I am told it was "my fault" I got pregnant, so I shouldn't expect special treatment, yet the same people believe they have the right to tell me what I should and shouldn't be doing while I am pregnant!!

Melissa, Lincoln, NE.

Bed Rest

I was on bed rest the last month and a half of my pregnancy due to an incompetent cervix. We have three dogs that demand a lot of attention, and they couldn't seem to understand why I wouldn't get up and walk them or play. My husband was out to sea for six weeks, so thank goodness for my in-laws. They came to stay and take care of me and my doggies. All I can say is I read a lot of books, watched a lot of TV, and ate a lot of snacks.

Ginger, Fort Collins, CO.

My doctor put me on bed rest for high blood pressure and severe headaches. I also had Gestational Diabetes. I was miserable, bored, lonely, eating all the time, and I couldn't wait to deliver! I put together photo albums, wrote letters to everyone I know out-of-town, and constantly thought about the baby's room. I wasn't going to get to decorate it like I had hoped.

Jillian, Chesterfield, MO.

My last month, my doctor put me on bed rest for pre-eclampsia. I kept going into labor at 34 and a half weeks. They thought he would only be 4 ½ pounds, but he surprised everyone (except me) by being big for his gestational age, 6 ½ pounds!!!

Kira, New Braunfels, TX.

In-Laws

My In-laws are wonderful. My mother-in-law nursed all five of her babies. She doesn't get weird when I'm in labor. With my first, I went to their house six hours after birth because my husband was working long hours in town. She did nice things for me but didn't "wait on me hand and foot." That would have bothered me. She encouraged me to eat and drink good things and stay healthy, but she wasn't pushy. She didn't take over the baby care but watched when I was nervous and told me how wonderful I was doing when I know I must have looked pretty funny trying to nurse. She held the baby when I took a shower and while I ate. She was just so comfortable with it all. My mother, on the other hand, is another story.

Tracy, Marietta, GA.

I said that as the baby's mom, it was my decision about whether or not to breastfeed my son, and that she should not tell me what I should do. My husband was mortified over the situation and said absolutely nothing. Afterward, he defended his mom by saying, "that's just the way my mom is." We had a major argument over that one. My relationship with my mother-in-law has been strained ever since (this was six years ago).

Gwen, Glendale, CA.

Maternity Leave

This was going to be our first baby, and I was able to take 12 weeks off work for maternity leave. It was sad thinking that 12 weeks would end, and I would have to take the little one to daycare every day. She would be there for eight hours a day, and I felt like someone else would be raising her. I would miss out on so much, and they wouldn't cherish little events like I would. I had to go back to work because we couldn't survive on my husband's income alone. I searched my brain trying to think of some at-home business I could do but found that seemed scary and inconsistent.

Morgan, Winchester, KY.

I never missed any time at work normally, but at six months began taking days off here and there. I felt guilty about it, but I was always so tired. The company I work for has been in existence for a long time, and I was only the second person ever to take maternity leave. It is a male dominated environment, and pregnancy problems were just something they didn't want to hear about. I got 18 weeks plus two weeks holiday entitlement, and my promotion was put on hold until I returned. If I could afford it, I would have stayed home with my little one instead.

Leah, Somers Point, NJ.

With my first two children, I took six months maternity leave and then went back to work full time. Fortunately I have my mother to watch my children, which has made my life less worrisome. With the latest addition, I decided to look into the possibility of working a three-day work week, so I could keep my benefits. My company offers a three or four day work week and job share.

Tabby, Bradenton, FL.

I work full-time and had to take my vacation as maternity leave and then go without pay for whatever other days I missed. My job is the sole source of income for my family and the only source of insurance. The one thing I have going for me is that my husband is a great stay at home dad, and probably does a better job than I would. I resented the fact that I couldn't be home more, but it all worked itself out.

Shawna, Tucson, AZ.

Nesting

I didn't notice my need to straighten the house and organize everything, but I noticed my husband did. I think he was nesting for me. I think the ninth month was the most nerve-wracking for him. As I would lie on the bed at night watching television, he would run around the house cleaning, putting things away, arranging baby clothes, and scrubbing what he had scrubbed the night before. I felt sort of guilty but not enough to do anything about it. I kind of liked the switch.

Lily, Houston, TX.

In my last month, my nesting instincts were the worst. I scrubbed walls, cleaned closets, re-organized my canned goods, and washed behind the washer and dryer and the oven. One night when I was supposed to be going to sleep with my husband, I jumped out of bed, went into the nursery and rearranged all the baby's hygiene products and hung some of her little outfits on hangers. My husband came in, looked at me, and he said, "you're definitely nesting honey." I didn't even realize how bad I had gotten until that night. Well, at least my baby would come home to a clean or immaculate home!

Laney, Albany, CA.

I have to say that my wife was acting like the Queen of England was coming to stay with us. I never complained, unless she was running me over with the vacuum. I actually liked her waiting on me and cleaning incessantly. What I thought was funny was the way she would put things back after she cleaned, and how I had to look forever to find what I needed.

Mark, Marion, OH.

Packing a Bag

Here's my list I used: Birth plan, telephone list, CD players and CDs, two pillows, rolling pin (works great for your back!), cards, vitamin E oil, hair scrunchies, 3 tubes of lip balm, overnight pads, 5 pairs of socks and panties, old, tattered robe with matching slippers, nursing gown, 2 of husband's T-shirts, Jello, granola bars, canned fruit, suckers, stretch pants and button down shirt for ride home. I also took waterproof mascara, a compact, lipstick, a sample of shampoo and conditioner, and Cranberry aromatherapy lotion.

Erin, Altus, OK.

With my first child, I packed everything that any list suggested, and I ended up using virtually none of it. Everyone is different, and you'll know if you need to bring the things suggested in books. Plus, if you don't pack something and need it, your husband or friend/family member can pick it up for you. Many hospitals also provide some things for your use. Here are some examples of things I didn't use: sugarless candy (hated it, popped one in my mouth and almost gagged), thick socks/slippers (have hot feet anyway), CDs and headset (too busy trying to have the baby, plus my husband had the TV on the whole time), playing cards (again, too busy having baby), snacks (can't eat them anyway and hospital has those too), and extra nightgowns and underwear (2 would probably be enough; I ended up wearing the hospital gowns. There is a lot to think about, and next time, I'll pack conservatively.

Maryanne, Scranton, PA.

Lists you find in books and magazines suggesting items you should take to the hospital with you are good in that they have great suggestions. However, I didn't take nearly as many things as many lists suggest. I wore elastic waist pants and over-sized T-shirts because people were coming in and out of my room so much. I should have packed more socks, since I love wearing them anyway. I did take all the necessary toiletries and such. But, I didn't take much else. I knew I wouldn't be playing cards with a baby in my arms. I knew I didn't care much for packing in the first place, so stuff like snacks didn't make it in. I did take nursing pads since I knew I'd start leaking the minute I didn't have them. The hospital provided most other stuff like sanitary pads, towels, and such.

Danielle, Ossining, NY.

Panic

About a week before my due date, I found myself in the baby's room thinking that I don't know the first thing about raising or taking care of a baby. After about 15 minutes of real panic, my husband calmed me down. After all, it was a little late to be worrying about that. Then, I began feeling like all of a sudden I was in a hurry to get ready and get everything I needed for the baby. Boy, looking back, I sure was neurotic that last month.

Kelly, Kihei, HI.

I was 21 and scared out of my mind. I had never in all of my life felt so out of control. I knew that there was this wonderful new life growing inside me and sometimes couldn't believe it was true. I was so emotional the whole time and would cry over the simplest things. With everything I experienced during my pregnancy, the crabbiness, the painful body changes, the insomnia, back aches, etc., I just didn't think the labor would go well and feared the worst. I really wasn't sure I could go through with it, but I couldn't see another choice. Talk about confused and scared.

Christy, Etters, PA.

I kept thinking to myself, "what if the tests were defective…what if there really is something wrong with the baby, or me?" I could come up with a million things to be scared about. I was scared and new to the whole idea of being pregnant and being a mom. I wanted the pregnancy so much, but I didn't know what to do next or if I'd know what to do in the future. Usually I am so strong, but there were moments around the end where I was so tired of being pregnant but scared of becoming a mom.

Donna, Roy, UT.

I really had no idea what to expect. I was scared out of my mind, and looking back, I didn't want my wife to know that. I questioned everything, especially my own talent as a father. Was I going to be able to handle the new baby? I didn't know how to change diapers, make bottles, or even hold a baby. It has taken me a long time to finally admit to my wife my feelings about her first pregnancy, and now I'm a seasoned pro with three wonderful kids. Fear is a natural part of becoming a father, something more women seem to instinctively understand.

Brian, Chicago.

Recipes for Home Inducing

I was miserable in my ninth month and was so ready to have my baby. I was told by a friend, and I read about this in a magazine, to drink raspberry tea. She and the magazine said it would produce a baby by making your contractions come on. Well, it didn't work for me, and I drank it every day for a week; although I did hear stories of other women who it did work for.

Angela T., Marshall, MN.

I remember hearing from a friend who was pregnant that riding down a bumpy road would bring on labor. I heard this could break your water. So, for the first two weeks of my ninth month, I drove down this really bumpy dirt road by my house. Nothing. I figured the baby wasn't ever going to come out!

Tina, Winston-Salem, NC.

I was complaining to my husband one night that I was totally ready for the baby to hurry up and be born so I wouldn't be so uncomfortable anymore. I was telling him all the things my co-workers had told me that might bring on contractions. I didn't feel like driving down a bumpy road and instead tried to get him to have sex. He hadn't really been into having sex nearly the whole time I was pregnant saying he thought it might hurt the baby. Well, I begged and begged (which is a first for me) and finally he gave in. I felt bad afterward about making him do it since it wasn't the greatest for either of us, and I never did have contractions afterward.

Melanie S., Hopewell, NJ.

I was a week late with my second baby, and I was miserable. I was talking to my mother, who always had advice, and she told me to hang curtains! I really didn't feel like doing this, but I kept thinking about it all that night. The next day nesting must have set in because I took all the curtains down in my house, washed them and pressed them and hung them back. I was exhausted. The following night, I was in the hospital having a baby.

Jackie, Egg Harbor, NJ.

Shopping

Around my last month, my husband and I bought a second-hand crib and changing table for $100, which brand new in the store would have cost us $1,000. I couldn't believe the prices of baby furniture. I just figured, why pay so much money when there's a good deal out there. When you add up the rest of the stuff like diapers, clothes, blankets, toys, you could end up spending your life savings.

Holly, Woodhaven, NY.

My husband and I decided to go baby shopping (at your normal everyday places) and couldn't believe the stuff and the prices! I found a cute furniture set we both loved. The girl spent 20 minutes explaining all the perks of the crib and dresser/ changing table trying to convince us. Then, she showed us the price. It was $750 for the crib and $950 for the dresser!! I almost had the baby right there and then. With all the other stuff we planned to buy, I felt out of my element.

Glenda, Kent, WA.

Old Wives Tales

When the baby is due, an apple will fall from a tree indicating that the baby, as the apple, is ripe.

If you had an easy/hard pregnancy, you will have a laid back / difficult child.

If you lie on your back frequently, the baby will stick to your back. Also, you will experience back labor during delivery.

Conclusions

In Closing

Help Coping with Pregnancy

This book is ending when the excitement is only beginning! The baby must be delivered and will be beginning a new life with you, and that's precisely why this book is ending! I'm saving the labor stories for another stack of pages. Those are always the longest, most interesting, and sometimes scariest stories. Look for *Labors Collected* and *The First Year Collected* to come behind this book soon.

The stories in this book are original, unique and shared. We are all looking for some company while struggling through life's unexpected turns, and pregnancy can be a serious matter that requires humor to survive through. Almost every pregnant woman can relate to these stories and a million others that long to be told.

I want to thank every one who took part in this book, the women who've shared their experiences with us all. If you'd like to share your story, email me at *CherylJProtin@msn.com*. I'd also like to thank my husband and my babies for bearing with me through this project. Thanks!

Keep reading for some great baby shower games!

Baby Shower Games

"Why is it that people rejoice at a birth and grieve at a funeral? It is because we are not the people involved."

—Mark Twain

The fun part is here, the celebration of a new life by gift and advice-giving, showing off a huge tummy, discussing the ins and outs of new motherhood, and most of all, playing games!! I thought I'd just throw in some of the best baby shower games I've seen over the years. I'm sure there are many more out there. Enjoy!

The Baby Quiz

Ask the baby's grandparents to write up what the parents were like as babies. Have them include vital statistics such as time of birth, weight, first smile, first tooth, age when toilet trained and early indications of personality. Based on this information, make up a quiz about the future parents to hand out to guests. The person with the most correct answers wins a prize!

Guess the Number of Jelly Beans in the Baby Bottle Game

Fill a baby bottle with little jelly beans (or other small candy, you can even get baby themed candy at some candy stores). Show the attendees the baby bottle and have them guess how many beans or candy are in the baby bottle. How about picking the mom's favorite small candy to use instead?

Also, use baby pins instead of candy in the guessing game for a low calorie version!

Treasure Hunt

Hide baby paraphernalia or small gifts around in the area where the shower is being held. Give the guests clues and a map, and have them search for the treasure. Depending on the number of guests, people can hunt individually or in teams.

Guess the Baby Food

Buy at least 10 different varieties of jar baby food. Label each with a number and write down each number with its contents on a piece of paper. Remove the food label, so the jar is now only recognizable by a number. Have your guests write down what they think is in each jar. The winner gets a prize.

Another variation is to have each guest put a sample of the baby food on a plate, write the number under the samples, and taste them. They then identify food based on its taste matching it to the number on the jar. Yuck or yum? I guess that depends!

Guess the Girth

You'll need a long and fairly wide piece of ribbon. Have your guests take turns writing their initials on the ribbon where they think represents the circumference of the mom-to-be's belly. After everyone has had a turn, the mother-to-be winds the ribbon around herself, and the person who was closest wins a prize.

Baby Picture Match Game

In advance, ask all the guests for pictures of themselves as babies. Assemble the photos on a board and assign each a number. At some point during the shower, pass out sheets of paper to the guests so they can match each baby to the appropriate grown-up. If the guests don't know each other well, give them nametags to wear. The person who gets the most correct answers wins.

Dress the Baby

Have a life-size baby doll, receiving blanket, cloth diaper, diaper wrap, and one-piece underwear. Write up a set of directions guests should follow. Then each guest should take turns trying to either dress or swaddle the baby. Time each guest. The one who does it the fastest wins. Fun!

Rock A Bye Baby

This game is like musical chairs or hot potato. The attendees stand in a circle with one holding a small baby doll. The mother-to-be sings a lullaby and each guest rocks the baby and then passes the baby on. When the mother-to-be stops singing the attendee holding the doll is out. Be sure to have each attendee rock the baby and throwing is not allowed! Funny!

Baby Bingo

Each guest should receive a paper that has 16 to 20 squares on it. Prior to the mother-to-be opening up the gifts, each guest puts down on their sheet what presents will be received (each square must be different). Each gift is then opened, and if you had written it in a square, you put an "X" through it. When you have all "X"'s crossed out diagonally, straight up or down or straight across, you win.

Balloon Carry

Place two laundry baskets across the room from each other, one with about 10 party balloons. Divide guests into two teams. Each member of the team puts a balloon between her knees and waddles across the room placing the balloon in the other laundry basket without touching the balloon with their hands. (Shaking, wiggling and hopping over the basket to free the balloon are all allowed!) The balloons get staticy so this can be tricky. After the attendee gets his/her balloon in the basket or drop it on the floor, he/she runs back and the next team member goes. Two teams can go at the same time with four baskets or one team at a time. Whichever team gets the most balloons in the basket within a certain time frame wins. This game is good for belly grabbing laughter especially if mom-to-be gets an honorary turn.

Remembering Baby Items on a Tray Game

Place several baby items on a tray. Present the tray to the attendees for 15 seconds. Then hide the tray and have them write down the baby items they remember. The baby shower attendee with the most correct items wins! The tray is then given to the guest of honor since she will need the items.

One variation is instead of putting the items on a tray, but them in a bag (do not use anything sharp) and let each attendee feel in the bag.

Another variation is to have one of the attendees dress up in footie pajamas and pin items/packages on them. The attendee carries a stuffed animal, bottle, etc. and parades around the room for a limited time. Everyone is so busy laughing that it is hard to remember anything!

Here are some sample items:

Baby Pins	Baby Shampoo	Travel Baby Oil	Ear syringe
Tweezers	Rattle	Cotton Balls	Syrup of Ipecac
Pair of socks	Small baby toys	Wash cloth	Small bottle/sipper

Try Not to Say "Baby" Game

Every baby shower attendee gets a baby diaper pin to pin on his/her clothes. Everyone tries not to say "Baby" during the party. When someone does, the first person who catches the slip, gets to confiscate the pin. The one with the most pins at the end of the party, wins!

Another variation on this game that is also used for Bridal Showers is to confiscate the pin when someone crosses his/her legs. This works best for smaller showers where everyone is sitting around a living room and can watch each other's legs!

Instead of using a pin, make candy pacifiers to put on a ribbon and wear around the neck. To make the pacifier, glue two white lifesavers together with one standing up on the other. Then glue one small jelly bean on the upright lifesaver. String the ribbon through the hole to make the necklace. If you use a peppermint or wintergreen lifesavers, then you get a pleasant smell. Cute!

Father-To-Be (Can't leave out Dad!)

The father-to-be places a balloon under his shirt with his birth weight listed on it. Everyone tries to guess the father-to-be's birth weight. He reads through the cards and then "gives birth" and the one who guesses the closest wins.

About the Author

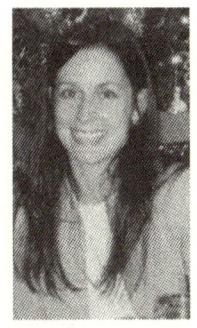

Cheryl Jean (Protin) Hancock began her writing career at the age of twelve writing poetry, short stories and songs for her own enjoyment and has kept with it ever since. A graduate of The University of Georgia, Mrs. Hancock is an English teacher in Athens, Georgia where she lives with her two beautiful children, Mara, age three and Derek, age nine. It was her love of her children and her personal experience of searching bookshelves for a better knowledge of her pregnancies that prompted her to write this book and make available to readers her and others' experiences. "Pregnancy can be frightening, but in here, you have friends." Mrs. Hancock is also the author of two career manuals published by Random House's LearningExpress. She states, "It is my love of writing that keeps me alive, no matter my subject matter."

www.ingramcontent.com/pod-product-compliance
Lightning Source LLC
Chambersburg PA
CBHW020252290526
45784CB00003B/1214